NCRP REPORT No. 145

Radiation Protection in Dentistry

Recommendations of the NATIONAL COUNCIL ON RADIATION PROTECTION AND MEASUREMENTS

Issued December 31, 2003

National Council on Radiation Protection and Measurement
7910 Woodmont Avenue, Suite 400 / Bethesda, MD 20814

LEGAL NOTICE

Library of Congress Cataloging-in-Publication Data

Radiation protection in dentistry / National Council on Radiation Protection and Measurements.
p. cm. -- (NCRP report ; no. 145)
"December 2003."
"This Report was prepared by Scientific Committee 91-2 on Radiation Protection in Dentistry."
Includes bibliographical references and index.
ISBN 0-929600-81-9
1. Teeth--Radiography--Safety measures. 2. Radiation--Safety measures. I. National Council on Radiation Protection and Measurements. II. Series.
RK309.R2725 2003
617.6'07572--dc22

2003027119

[For detailed information on the availability of NCRP publications see page 174.]

Preface

This Report was developed under the auspices of Scientific Committee 91, the National Council on Radiation Protection and Measurements' (NCRP) program area committee concerned with radiation protection in medicine. The Report provides radiation protection guidance for the use of x rays in dental practice, including advice on shielding design for dental x-ray facilities. It supersedes NCRP Report No. 35, Dental X-Ray Protection, which was issued in March 1970.

The Report is dedicated to the memory of George W. Casarett, Ph.D., former Professor of Radiation Biology and Biophysics at the University of Rochester School of Medicine and Dentistry, for his enduring contributions to the NCRP, radiation biology, and radiation health sciences communities, and for his incomparable scientific, scholarly and graceful mentoring of dentists in the radiation sciences.

This Report was prepared by Scientific Committee 91-2 on Radiation Protection in Dentistry. Serving on Scientific Committee 91-2 were:

Co-Chairmen

John W. Brand
University of Detroit Mercy School of Dentistry
Detroit, Michigan

S. Julian Gibbs
Vanderbilt University Medical Center
Nashville, Tennessee

Members

Marc Edwards
Radiation Oncology Associates of Kansas City
Overland Park, Kansas

Alan G. Lurie
University of Connecticut School of Dental Medicine
Farmington, Connecticut

Jerald O. Katz
University of Missouri-Kansas City School of Dentistry
Kansas City, Missouri

Stuart C. White
University of California-Los Angeles School of Dentistry
Los Angeles, California

Consultant
W. Doss McDavid
University of Texas Health Science Center
San Antonio, Texas

NCRP Secretariat
Marvin Rosenstein, *Consultant,* 2001-2003
Thomas M. Koval, *Senior Staff Scientist,* 1998-2000
James A. Spahn, Jr., *Senior Staff Scientist,* 1995-1998
Cindy L. O'Brien, *Managing Editor*

The Council wishes to express its appreciation to the Committee members for the time and effort devoted to the preparation of this Report.

Thomas S. Tenforde
President

Contents

1. Introduction

Radiology is an essential component of dental diagnosis. Available data clearly show that ionizing radiation, if delivered in sufficient doses, may produce biological damage. However, it is not clear that radiation in doses required for dental radiography presents any risk. Neither is it clear that these small doses are free of risk. The practitioner may reasonably expect that the health benefit to the patient from dental radiographic examination will outweigh any potential risk from radiation exposure provided that:

- the dental radiographic examination is clinically indicated and justified
- the technique is optimized to ensure high-quality diagnostic images
- the principles outlined in this Report are followed to minimize exposure to the patient, staff and the public

Office design, equipment, and procedures that minimize patient exposure will also reduce exposure to the operator and the public. Additional measures, however, may be required to ensure that doses to operators and the public are within limits established by regulatory bodies. Doses to all should be kept as low as reasonably achievable, with economic and social factors being taken into account (*i.e.*, the ALARA principle) (NCRP, 1990). For operators and the public, the ALARA principle applies to further reduction of doses that are already below regulatory limits. The concept may be extended to patients for whom no regulatory limits exist. It states that all reasonable efforts should be made to reduce or eliminate avoidable radiation exposure, so long as scarce resources are not unduly diverted from other societal needs that may be more critical (NCRP, 1998).

1.1 Purpose

The objective of this Report is to present methods and procedures for radiation protection in the dental office. The goals are: (1) to eliminate unnecessary radiation exposure to the patient, *i.e.*, radiation not necessary to produce optimal quality radiographs; and (2) to ensure that exposures to office staff and the public are within recommended limits and meet the ALARA principle. This Report makes a number of recommendations for the dentist to achieve these goals.

1.2 Scope

This Report provides guidelines for radiation protection in the use of x rays in dental practice. It replaces the National Council on Radiation Protection and Measurements' (NCRP) Report No. 35 (NCRP, 1970) in its entirety. It presents recommendations regarding performance and optimal use of dental x-ray equipment, as well as recommendations for radiation protection surveys and monitoring of personnel. Sections are included for the specific guidance of dentists, their clinical associates, and qualified experts conducting radiation protection surveys, calibration procedures, equipment performance evaluations, and determining facility shielding and layout designs. Also included is guidance for equipment designers, manufacturers, and service personnel. Basic guidance for dentists and their office staff is contained in the body; technical details are provided in the appendices. Certain aspects of radiation protection unique to dental radiology (*e.g.*, the impact of infection control measures on radiation protection) are included (Appendix A).

Since the target audience may not have easy access to related documents, this Report is intended to be a stand-alone document, providing sufficient background and guidance for most applications. Additional details may be found in other reports of the NCRP (1976; 1988; 1989a; 1989b; 1990; 1992; 1993a; 1993b; 1997; 1998; 2000; 2001; in press). Further, the intent is to focus on those radiographic procedures commonly performed in dental facilities, especially intraoral, panoramic and cephalometric dental radiographic equipment and techniques. Except as otherwise specified, the recommendations in this Report apply to these procedures. Other procedures of oral and maxillofacial radiology that are not generally practiced in the dental office, and that require more sophisticated equipment, are subject to the requirements and recommendations for medical radiology (NCRP, 1989a; 1989b; 2000) and will not be specifically addressed in this Report.

1.3 Radiation Protection Philosophy

Biological effects of ionizing radiation fall into two classes: deterministic and stochastic (Appendix B). Deterministic effects occur in all individuals who receive a high dose, *i.e.*, exceeding some threshold. Examples of these effects are acute radiation sickness, cataract, and epilation. Their severity is proportional to dose, implying the presence of a threshold dose below which no clinically-significant effects occur. Stochastic effects, such as cancer, are all-or-nothing effects. That is, either a radiation-induced cancer occurs or it does not; its severity is not dose dependent. The probability of its occurrence is proportional to dose, implying the absence of a threshold. The basic goal of radiation protection is to prevent in exposed individuals the occurrence of deterministic effects and to reduce the potential for stochastic effects to an acceptable level when benefits of that exposure are considered (NCRP, 1993a). Achievement of this goal requires two interrelated activities: (1) efforts to ensure that no individual receives a dose greater than the recommended limit and (2) efforts to ensure that doses are ALARA. In most applications, ALARA is simply the continuation of good radiation protection programs and practices that have traditionally been effective in keeping the average of individual exposures of monitored workers well below the limits. Cost-benefit analysis is applied to measures taken to achieve ALARA goals. For each source or type of radiation exposure, it is determined whether the benefits outweigh the costs. Second, the relation of cost to benefit from the reduction or elimination of that exposure is evaluated. Frequently costs and benefits are stated in disparate units. Costs may be in units such as adverse biological effects or economic expenditure. Benefits may be in units such as disease detected or lives saved. Three principles provide the basis for all actions taken for purposes of radiation protection. They are:

1. Justification: The benefit of radiation exposure outweighs any accompanying risk.
2. Optimization: Total exposure remains as low as reasonably achievable, with economic and social factors taken into account (the ALARA principle).
3. Dose limitation: Dose limits are applied to each individual to ensure that no one is exposed to an unacceptably high risk.

All three of these principles are applied to evaluation of occupational and public exposure. The first two apply to exposure of patients. However, no dose limit is established for diagnostic or therapeutic exposure of patients. The primary objective is to ensure that the health benefit overrides the risk to the patient from that exposure.

NCRP has established recommended dose limits for occupational and public exposure (Table 1.1) (NCRP, 1993a). Limits have been set below the estimated human threshold doses for deterministic effects. NCRP assumes that for radiation protection purposes, the risk of stochastic effects is proportional to dose without threshold, throughout the range of dose and dose rates of importance in routine radiation protection (NCRP, 1993a). This principle was used to set dose limits for occupationally-exposed individuals such that estimated risks of stochastic effects are no greater than risks of occupational injury in other vocations that are generally regarded as safe (Table 1.2).

TABLE 1.1—*Recommended dose limits (NCRP, 1993a).*[a]

Basis	Dose Limit
	Occupational
Stochastic effects	50 mSv annual effective dose 10 mSv × age (y) cumulative effective dose
Deterministic effects	150 mSv annual equivalent dose to lens of eye 500 mSv annual equivalent dose to skin, hands and feet
	Public
Stochastic effects	1 mSv annual effective dose for continuous or frequent exposure 5 mSv annual effective dose for infrequent exposure
Deterministic effects	15 mSv annual equivalent dose to lens of eye 50 mSv annual equivalent dose to skin, hands and feet
Embryo and fetus	0.5 mSv equivalent dose in a month from occupational exposure of the mother once pregnancy is known

[a]The appropriate dose limits for adult students (*i.e.*, age 18 or older) in dental, dental hygiene, and dental assisting educational programs depend on whether the educational entity classifies the student as occupationally exposed or not. Additional guidance for radiation protection practices for educational institutions is given in NCRP (1966). Dose limits for students under 18 y of age are given in NCRP (1993a), and correspond to the limits for members of the public.

Two terms used in this Report have a special meaning as indicated by the use of italics:

1. ***Shall* and *shall not* are used to indicate that adherence to the recommendation is considered necessary to meet accepted standards of protection.**
2. ***Should* and *should not* are used to indicate a prudent practice to which exceptions may occasionally be made in appropriate circumstances.**

The use of ionizing radiation in the healing arts is a well-regulated activity in the United States. The federal government has established a performance standard that controls manufacture and installation of x-ray generating equipment designed for clinical use (FDA, 1995). The states (or other political jurisdictions) have implemented regulations that govern users, including dentists. These regulations pertain to design of facilities, especially radiation shielding, as well as use and maintenance of equipment.

TABLE 1.2—*Fatal accident rates, United States, 1991 (NCRP, 1993a).*

Industry Group	Fatality Rate (per 10,000 workers per year)
Trade	0.4
Manufacturing	0.4
Service	0.4
Government	0.9
Radiation	0.2 – 2.0[a]
Transportation, public utilities	2.2
Construction	3.1
Mining, quarrying	4.3
Agriculture	4.4
All groups	0.9

[a]Lifetime fatal cancer risk from each year's exposure (assuming a risk coefficient of 4×10^{-2} Sv^{-1}, and occupational effective doses to an average worker between 0.5 and 5 mSv y^{-1}). Estimated using the linear nonthreshold model. Actual fatal cancer risk for radiation may be more, less, or even zero. Entries for other industries are taken from actuarial data for fatal work-related accidents.

Dentists *shall* use x-ray equipment and procedures in a manner that ensures compliance with both the recommendations in this Report and the requirements of their state or political jurisdictions. When there are discrepancies between these recommendations and legal requirements, the more rigorous *shall* take precedence.

2. General Considerations

All persons are exposed to radiation in their daily lives (NCRP, 1987a; 1987b; 1987c; 1989c; 1989d). NCRP has estimated the mean effective dose equivalent from all sources in the United States as 3.6 mSv y^{-1} (Figure 2.1). Approximately 3 mSv of this arises from

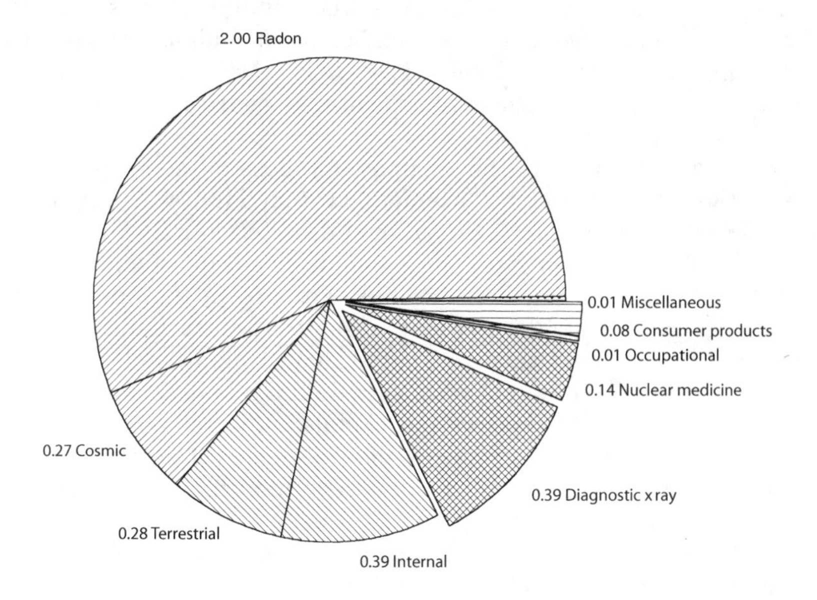

Fig. 2.1. U.S. average annual effective dose equivalent (per capita) from all sources in 1987. The total (rounded) is 3.6 mSv y^{-1}. About 3 mSv of this is from naturally-occurring sources: 2 mSv from inhalation of radon and its radioactive decay products; 0.27 mSv from cosmic radiation; 0.28 mSv from radioactive materials in our surrounding earth, building materials, etc.; and 0.39 mSv from radioactive sources within our bodies. Most man-made radiation comes from diagnostic exposure in the healing arts (~0.5 mSv), with small quantities from occupational sources, consumer products such as smoke detectors or luminous watch dials, and miscellaneous sources such as cosmic radiation exposure during air travel as a passenger (NCRP, 1987b).

naturally-occurring sources; these sources have been present since the beginning of the Earth. Only 0.6 mSv comes from man-made sources, most of which is from diagnostic exposure in the healing arts. Recent data from Switzerland indicate that dental x rays contribute approximately one percent of the total dose from the healing arts (Aroua *et al.*, 2002). Thus, dental radiation is a minor contributor to total population burden. However, appropriate measures are necessary to maintain dental radiation exposures ALARA.

2.1 Dose Limits

The Council has recommended annual and cumulative dose limits for individuals from occupational radiation exposure, and separate annual dose limits for members of the public from sources of man-made radiation (Table 1.1) (NCRP, 1993a). The dose limits do not apply to diagnostic or therapeutic exposure of the patient in the healing arts.

The cumulative limit for occupational dose is more restrictive than the annual limit. For example, an individual who begins at age 18 to receive annual occupational doses of 50 mSv will in 4 y receive 200 mSv, approaching the cumulative limit of 220 mSv at age 22. At that point, occupational exposure to that individual would be confined by the cumulative, not the annual limit. That is, the individual would then be limited to a cumulative dose at the average rate of 10 mSv y^{-1}, with a maximum rate of 50 mSv in any 1 y. Occupationally-exposed individuals may be monitored for work-related radiation exposure and the duties of any individual who approaches the annual or cumulative limit may be changed so the limit is not exceeded.

Since members of the public do not wear monitors, facilities are designed, operated and monitored such that no individual can receive a dose in excess of the recommended limit.

Published data indicate that average dental occupational exposures are usually only a small fraction of the limit and are less than most other workers in the healing arts (Table 2.1) (Kumazawa *et al.*, 1984). Occupational exposures have been declining (Figure 2.2) over recent decades in workers in both the healing arts in general and dentistry in particular (HSE, 1998; Kumazawa *et al.*, 1984; UNSCEAR, 2000). It seems reasonable to conclude that no dental personnel will receive occupational exposures exceeding the limit unless there are problems with facility design, equipment performance, or operating procedures.

TABLE 2.1—*Occupational doses in the healing arts, United States, 1980.*[a]

Occupational Subgroup	Number of Workers		Mean Annual Whole-Body Dose (mSv)	
	Total[b]	Exposed[c]	Total[b]	Exposed[c]
Hospital	126,000	86,000	1.4	2.0
Medical offices	155,000	87,000	1.0	1.8
Dental	259,000	82,000	0.2	0.7
Podiatry	8,000	3,000	0.1	0.3
Chiropractic	15,000	6,000	0.3	0.8
Veterinary	21,000	12,000	0.6	1.1
Total	584,000	276,000	0.7	1.5

[a]Kumazawa *et al.* (1984).
[b]All workers with potential occupational exposure.
[c]Workers who received a measurable dose in any monitoring period during the year.

No individual *shall* be permitted to receive an occupational effective dose in excess of 50 mSv in any 1 y. The numerical value of the individual worker's lifetime occupational effective dose *shall* be limited to 10 mSv times the value of his or her age in years.

Occupational equivalent dose *shall not* exceed 0.5 mSv in a month to the embryo or fetus for pregnant individuals, once pregnancy is known.

Mean nonoccupational effective dose to frequently or continuously exposed members of the public *shall not* exceed 1 mSv y^{-1} (excluding doses from natural background and medical care); infrequently exposed members of the public *shall not* be exposed to effective doses greater than 5 mSv in any year.

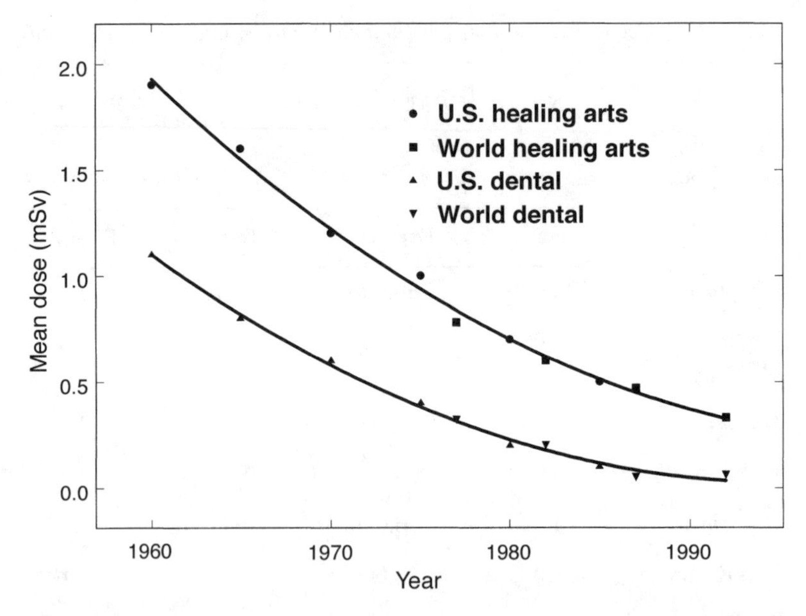

Fig. 2.2. Decline in mean occupational doses over recent decades, for workers in all healing arts combined and dentistry. United States data at 5 y intervals from 1960 to 1980 plus that projected for 1985 were reported as dosimeter readings (Kumazawa *et al.*, 1984). World estimates from 1975 to 1995 were reported as effective doses and are plotted at each 5 y interval (UNSCEAR, 2000). Dental workers do not generally wear leaded aprons, so differences between dosimeter readings and effective doses may be small (Appendix C).

Dental facility design, x-ray equipment performance and operating procedures *shall* be such that no individual exposure exceeds these recommended dose limits.

Facility design, x-ray equipment performance and operating procedures *should* be established to maintain patient, occupational and public exposures as low as reasonably achievable, economic and social factors being taken into account (the ALARA principle).

The ALARA principle is an optimization of radiation protection concept applied to each facility. Thus it imposes no numeric limitations of effective dose below the established effective dose limits (Table 1.1). The goal is that the entire radiology operation be designed to reduce radiation exposure to the minimum achievable for the specific facility without incurring undue cost or compromising patient care. That is, effective doses achieved through application of the ALARA principle may vary by facility or even by specific x-ray machine in a given facility. In dentistry, the application of the ALARA principle is expected to reduce effective doses to individuals well below the applicable dose limits.

2.2 Role of Dental Personnel in Radiation Protection

ALARA requires optimizing the practices of all dental personnel that are involved in prescription, exposure, processing, evaluation and interpretation of dental radiographs. This Section describes the roles of each.

2.2.1 *The Dentist*

In most dental facilities, the dentist in charge is responsible for the design and conduct of the radiation protection program (NRPB, 2001). In large facilities, such as dental educational institutions, the authority and responsibility for design and oversight of the radiation protection program may be delegated to a specific employee with special expertise in the field. This individual is designated the radiation safety officer. The dentist in charge, in consultation with the radiation safety officer (if that person is someone other than the dentist) and with a qualified expert, is responsible for implementing the radiation protection program, which includes (NCRP, 1990; 1998):

- establishing, reviewing and documenting radiation protection procedures
- instructing staff in radiation protection
- implementing radiation surveys and recording results and corrective actions
- establishing the monitoring of personnel, if required
- ensuring that all radiation protection features are functional and the required warning signs are posted
- implementing and monitoring the ALARA principle
- implementing and documenting quality-assurance procedures

The dentist (or, in some facilities, the designated radiation safety officer) *shall* establish a radiation protection program as outlined above. The dentist *shall* seek guidance of a qualified expert in this activity.

The dentist is qualified by education and licensure to prescribe and perform radiographic examinations and to process, evaluate and interpret the images produced.

All radiographic examinations *shall* be performed only on direct prescription of the dentist or physician. These procedures *shall* be prescribed only after conduct of a clinical history and physical examination of the patient, and determination of a reasonable expectation of a health benefit to the patient.

2.2.2 *Auxiliary Personnel*

In most dental facilities the staff involved in radiologic procedures consists of registered dental hygienists and of dental assistants who may or may not be certified. Registered hygienists and certified assistants are trained and credentialed to perform radiologic exposures, process the images and evaluate them for quality (NRPB, 2001). In some states noncertified assistants may be credentialed for these procedures upon completion of approved training.

Dental radiographic exposures *shall* be performed only by dentists or by legally qualified and credentialed auxiliary personnel. Opportunities *should* be provided for auxiliary personnel to attend appropriate continuing education courses.

2.2.3 *The Qualified Expert*

This individual is qualified by education and experience to perform advanced or complex procedures in radiation protection that generally are beyond the capabilities of most dental personnel (NRPB, 2001). These procedures include facility design to provide adequate shielding for protection of the occupationally exposed and the public, inspection and evaluation of performance of x-ray equipment, or evaluation and recommendation of radiation protection programs (including the ALARA principle). Generally possessing an advanced degree in medical physics, medical health physics, or a similar field, this individual is usually certified by the American Board of Radiology, the American Board of Medical Physics, American Board of Health Physics, or equivalent. Care must be taken to ensure that the qualified expert's credentials include knowledge and familiarity with dental radiologic practices. Some otherwise highly qualified experts may have little experience in dental radiological practices (Michel and Zimmerman, 1999). Some states credential or license these individuals. The principal responsibility of this person is to serve as a consultant to the dentist.

The dentist or designer *shall* obtain guidance of a qualified expert in the design of dental facilities and establishment of radiation protection policies and procedures.

3. Radiation Protection in Dental Facilities

Radiation protection recommendations specific to the dental facility are provided in this Section. Technical details are found in the appendices.

3.1 Protection of the Patient

Potential health benefits to patients from dental x-ray exposure preclude establishment of specific and meaningful dose limits for patients. Thus the specific goal of protection of the patient should be to obtain the required clinical information while avoiding unnecessary patient exposure.

3.1.1 *Examination Extent and Frequency*

Elimination of unnecessary radiographic examinations is a very effective measure for avoiding unnecessary patient exposure. Procedures are outlined in the following sections for eliminating unnecessary examinations for both symptomatic patients seeking urgent care and asymptomatic patients scheduled for routine or continuing dental care.

A clear procedure for reducing the extent and frequency of dental radiographic examinations needs to be followed when a patient transfers or is referred from one dentist to another. Modern digital imaging and electronic transfer facilitates exchange of information among dentists and other health care providers.

For each new or referred patient, the dentist *shall* make a good faith attempt to obtain recent, pertinent radiographs from the patient's previous dentist.

Radiographic examinations *shall* be performed only when indicated by patient history, physical examination by the dentist, or laboratory findings.

3.1.1.1 *Symptomatic Patients.* When symptomatic patients are seen, the dentist is obligated to provide care to relieve those symptoms and, when possible, eliminate their cause. Radiographs required for that treatment are fully justified, but additional noncontributory radiographs are not. For example, a full-mouth intraoral study is not warranted for emergency treatment of a single painful tooth. However, if treatment of that painful tooth is the first step in comprehensive dental care, then those radiographs required for that comprehensive care are justified.

For symptomatic patients, radiographic examination *shall* be limited to those images required for diagnosis and planned treatment (local or comprehensive) of current disease.

3.1.1.2 *Asymptomatic Patients.* Maintenance of oral health in asymptomatic new patients or those returning for periodic re-examination without clear signs and symptoms of oral disease may require radiographs. Selection criteria that will aid the dentist in selecting and prescribing radiographic examination of these patients have been published (Appendix D) (Joseph, 1987; Matteson, 1997; Matteson *et al.*, 1991). These criteria recommend that dental radiographs be prescribed only when the patient's history and physical findings suggest a reasonable expectation that radiographic examination will produce clinically useful information.

For asymptomatic patients, the extent of radiographic examination of new patients, and the frequency and extent for return patients, *should* adhere to published selection criteria.

3.1.1.3 *Administrative Radiographs.* Radiographs are occasionally requested, usually by outside agencies, for purposes other than health. Examples include requests from third-party payment agencies for proof of treatment or from regulatory boards to determine competence of the practitioner. In some institutions dental or dental auxiliary students have been required to perform oral radiographic examinations on other students for the sole purpose of learning the technique. Other methods (such as photographs for treatment documentation or image receptor and tubehead placement for radiologic technique training) that do not require exposure to x rays are generally available for providing this information.

Administrative use of radiation to provide information not related to health of the patient *shall not* be permitted. Students *shall not* be permitted to perform radiographic exposures of patients, other students, or volunteers solely for purposes of their education or licensure.

3.1.2 *Radiation Exposure per Image*

Patient exposure per intraoral film, measured at skin entry, has been reduced significantly since the early days of dental radiology (Figure 3.1). These reductions have been accomplished by improvements in x-ray equipment, operating procedures, and films. The total number of films exposed per year in the United States has increased at a rate faster than growth of the population (FDA, 1973; NCHCT, 1982; UNSCEAR, 2000). Continuing efforts are needed to provide further reduction of exposure per image. A method to achieve this goal is the use of a diagnostic reference level. A diagnostic reference level is a patient dose-related quantity per x-ray procedure or image that, if consistently exceeded in clinical practice, should elicit investigation and efforts for improved patient dose management (ICRP, 1996a; Napier, 1999). Suggested values of diagnostic reference levels at skin entry for common dental x-ray projections (bitewings and cephalometric) have been published (CRCPD, 2003; Gray *et al.*, in press; NRPB, 1999). The diagnostic reference levels in the United States are expressed as entrance skin exposure (in milliroentgens) or entrance air kerma (in milligray), and for bitewings are a function of film speed (*i.e.*, D-, E- or F-speed film) and operating potential (*i.e.*, 50 to 100 kVp) (CRCPD, 2003) (see Glossary for explanation of these quantities). A number of states have established diagnostic reference levels that are applicable for a given state (CRCPD, 2003). It is the responsibility of the dentist to choose the fastest available image receptor (direct-exposure film, screen film, or digital) (Appendix E) consistent with the imaging requirements of each specific examination.

3.1.3 *X-Ray Machines*

All x-ray machines need to meet the design specifications in Section 4 and all requirements of the jurisdiction in which they are located. Equipment certified to conform to the federal performance standard (FDA, 1995) will generally meet these requirements. Equipment of recent manufacture (especially that manufactured in

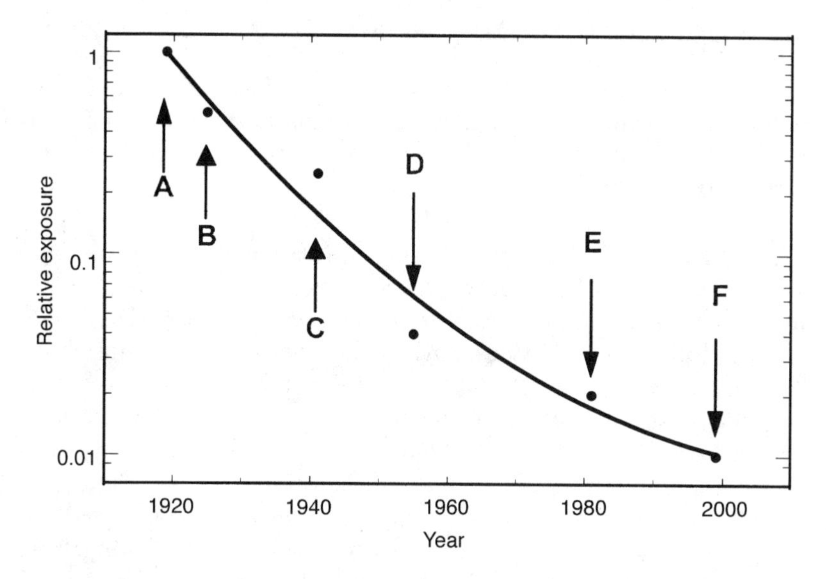

Fig. 3.1. Relative exposure at skin entry for intraoral radiographs, 1920 to 2000. Arrows indicate introduction of faster films (ANSI speed groups A, B, C, D, E, and F, as indicated). The exposure required for F-speed film is approximately one percent of that required for the first dental films (Farman and Farman, 2000).

Europe) also conforms to international standards (IEC, 1994; NRPB, 2001). Section 4 outlines parameters of equipment design; it provides guidance to manufacturers and may be useful to the dentist in selecting and purchasing x-ray machines. Portable x-ray equipment is intended for use with debilitated patients whose physical condition prevents transporting them to fixed radiographic facilities. It is not the purpose of portable x-ray equipment to provide for convenience of the operator or of healthy patients.

Personnel responsible for purchase and operation of dental x-ray equipment *shall* ensure that such equipment meets or exceeds all applicable governmental requirements and regulations, plus the design specifications summarized in Section 4. In addition, the equipment *should* conform to international standards.

Portable x-ray machines *shall not* be used when fixed installations are available and patients' conditions permit their use.

3.1.4 *Examinations and Procedures*

The general requirements and recommendations in this Report apply to all dental radiologic examinations and procedures. This Section, however, presents additional recommendations specific for particular radiographic examinations.

3.1.4.1 *Intraoral Radiography.* Dental intraoral radiographs and chest radiographs have been the most common diagnostic x-ray procedures in the United States (Brown *et al.*, 1980; FDA, 1973; Mettler, 1987). In both cases, patient dose per image is small; however, the number of such procedures performed annually requires diligence in optimizing the radiation exposure from procedures so that unnecessary exposure is avoided.

3.1.4.1.1 *Beam energy.* Dental x-ray machines have been marketed for intraoral radiography with operating potentials ranging from 40 to more than 100 kVp (kilovolt peak). However, the U.S. federal performance standard now requires that low-kVp (less than 60) intraoral dental x-ray machines be heavily filtered such that effective beam energies will approach that of 60 kVp machines (FDA, 1995). Published data show no significant relationship between operating potential and effective dose to the patient with beams ranging from 70 to 90 kVp (Gibbs *et al.*, 1988a). These data apply specifically to half-wave rectified dental x-ray machines. Similar beam energy spectra are produced by constant-potential machines operating some 10 kV below the kVp of these conventional machines. There is little to be gained from operating potentials higher than 80 kVp. Many contemporary machines operate at a fixed operating potential which, if in the 60 to 80 kVp range, is generally acceptable.

> **The operating potential of dental x-ray machines *shall not* be less than 50 kVp and *should not* be less than 60 kVp. Also, the operating potential *shall not* be more than 100 kVp and *should not* be more than 80 kVp.**

3.1.4.1.2 *Position-indicating device.* Pointed cones have been commonly used as position-indicating devices for aiming x-ray beams for intraoral radiography. However, they are not suitable for positive beam-receptor alignment (Section 4) and have been largely replaced with open-end parallel-wall devices that are either circular or rectangular in cross-section. These devices are not collimators. Thus, their inside dimensions are equal to or slightly larger than the dimensions of the beam at the position-indicating device tip. The position-indicating device may be lined with metal to absorb scattered radiation arising from the collimator and filter.

Position-indicating devices *shall* be open-ended devices with provision for attenuation of scattered radiation arising from the collimator or filter.

Short source-to-skin distances (or source-to-image receptor distances) produce unfavorable dose distributions (van Aken and van der Linden, 1966). They may degrade the sharpness of the images, and also produce excessive magnification or distortion of the image, sometimes limiting anatomic coverage.

Source-to-image receptor distance for intraoral radiography *shall not* be less than 20 cm and *should not* be less than 40 cm.

3.1.4.1.3 *Rectangular collimation.* Existing requirements and recommendations require that all medical and dental diagnostic x-ray procedures except intraoral radiography be performed with the beam collimated to the area of clinical interest; in no case can it be larger than the image receptor (FDA, 1995). Positive beam-receptor alignment is required to ensure that all exposed tissue is recorded on the image. However, requirements and recommendations to date have permitted circular beams for intraoral radiography whose area, measured in the plane of the receptor, may be up to five times the area of the receptor. Published data show that rectangular collimation of the beam to the size of the image receptor reduces the tissue volume exposed (Figure 3.2). This would reduce the effective dose to the patient by a factor of four to five, without adverse influence on image quality (Freeman and Brand, 1994; Gibbs, 2000; Gibbs *et al.*, 1988a; Underhill *et al.*, 1988). Effective devices for positive beam-receptor alignment for periapical radiography have been commercially available at nominal cost for many years, providing rectangular collimation for routine clinical use.

Beam-receptor alignment devices for conventional interproximal (bitewing) radiography remain only marginally effective. Conventional bitewing technique, with the long axis of the standard intraoral image receptor horizontal, requires that the teeth be in or very near occlusal contact during exposure, in order to provide required anatomic coverage including not only the crowns of the teeth but also the crestal alveolar bone. Two approaches have been devised: (1) paper bite tabs, thin enough to provide for sufficient

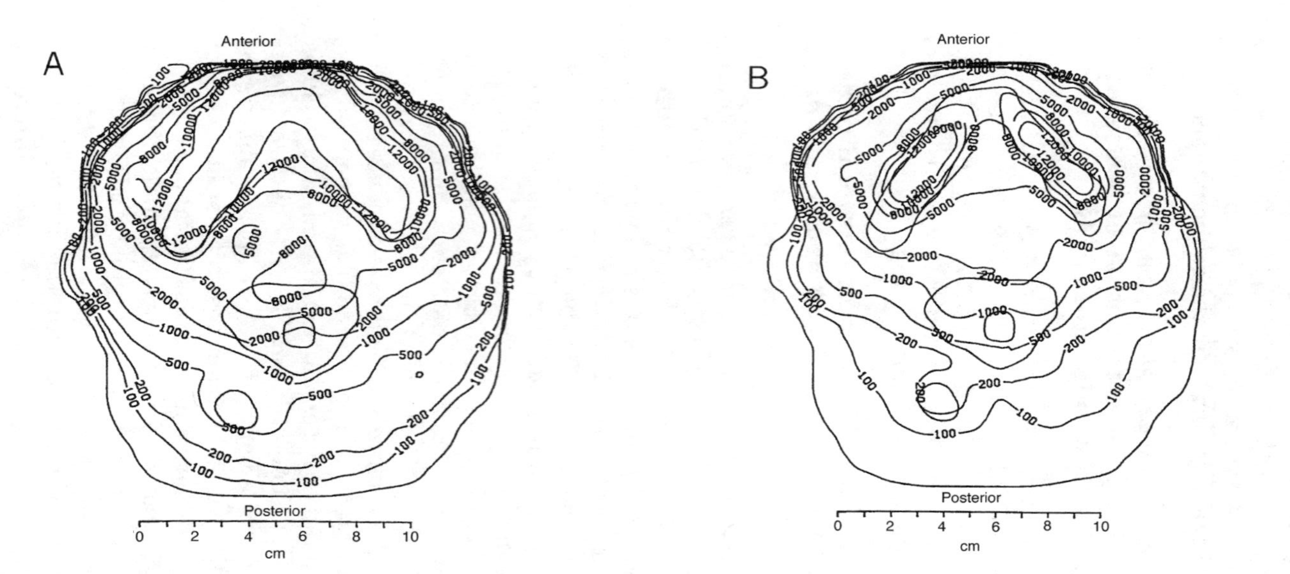

Fig. 3.2. Isodose curves calculated for full-mouth intraoral examinations obtained at 80 kVp using optimum exposures for D-speed film. Lines without numeric annotations indicate skin surface and internal hard tissue surfaces. Numeric annotations indicate absorbed dose in microgray (1,000 µGy = 1 mGy). For example, the tissues contained within the contour labeled 5,000 receive an absorbed dose of at least 5 mGy (5,000 µGy). (A) Transverse section through the occlusal plane, 7 cm round beams. Note that the teeth receive absorbed doses of at least 12 mGy, and all tissues anterior to the cervical spine receive at least 5 mGy. (B) Same plane with rectangular collimation. Areas contained within each isodose contour are smaller than in A. Absorbed dose is generally confined to the facial area, with posterior regions receiving absorbed doses no greater than 1 mGy (Gibbs *et al.*, 1987).

anatomic coverage but not sufficiently rigid and (2) plastic bite tabs, sufficiently rigid but too thick to allow desired anatomic coverage. This problem can be solved by placing the bitewing image receptor with the long axis oriented vertically.

Alternatively, a new image receptor size could be developed to provide bitewing images that include crestal bone, with the long axis of the image receptor oriented horizontally. In other words, rectangular collimation of the x-ray beam is available for periapical and vertical bitewing radiography; future developments may make it practical for other projections, including occlusal and horizontal bitewing. Perfect rectangular collimation, with the beam dimensions exactly equal to those of the image receptor, is difficult if not impossible to achieve. Tolerance in beam dimensions is allowable to reduce required precision of beam-receptor alignment to an accomplishable level.

Rectangular collimation of the x-ray beam *shall* be routinely used for periapical radiography. Each dimension of the beam, measured in the plane of the image receptor, *should not* exceed the dimension of the image receptor by more than two percent of the source-to-image receptor distance. Similar collimation *should* be used, when feasible, for interproximal (bitewing) radiography. Anatomy or the inability of occasional specific patients to cooperate, including some children, may make rectangular collimation and beam-receptor alignment awkward or impossible for some projections. The requirement may be relaxed in these rare cases.

Positive beam-receptor alignment allows more freedom in patient positioning. Many dentists prefer to recline the patient fully, rotating the head left or right, and maintaining the beam near vertical.

3.1.4.1.4 *Image receptor.* Since the mid-1950s the most common image receptor (Appendix E) for intraoral radiography in the United States has been direct-exposure film of American National Standards Institute (ANSI) Speed Group D (Goren *et al.*, 1989; Platin *et al.*, 1998). Faster films, ANSI Speed Group E, were introduced in the early 1980s, with improved versions coming in the mid-1990s. These faster films have been widely used in Europe (Svenson and Petersson, 1995; Svenson *et al.*, 1996). Published data show that these faster films provide for patient dose reductions of up to 50 percent. However, early E-speed films exhibited decreased contrast and higher sensitivity to processing conditions than was found with D-speed films (Diehl *et al.*, 1986; Thunthy and Weinberg, 1982). These problems have been corrected and current E-speed film can be used with no degradation of diagnostic information (Conover *et al.*, 1995; Hintze *et al.*, 1994; 1996; Kitagawa *et al.*, 1995; Nakfoor and Brooks, 1992; Price, 1995; Svenson *et al.*, 1997a; Tamburus and Lavrador, 1997; Tjelmeland *et al.*, 1998). Digital image receptors with speeds similar to or faster than E-speed film are available. Intraoral films of speed group F are commercially available. Initial data suggest suitability of these films for routine use (Farman and Farman, 2000; Ludlow *et al.*, 2001; Thunthy, 2000). If these results are confirmed, these films should be considered for routine use. Future developments are likely to include even faster films and digital receptors.

Image receptors of speeds slower than ANSI Speed Group E films *shall not* be used for intraoral radiography. Faster receptors *should* be evaluated and adopted if found acceptable.

3.1.4.1.5 *Patient restraint.* It may be necessary in some cases that uncooperative patients be restrained during exposure or that the image receptor be held in place by hand. A member of the patient's family (or other caregiver) provides this restraint or receptor retention.

Occupationally-exposed personnel *shall not* restrain uncooperative patients or hold the image receptor in place during an x-ray exposure. Members of the public who restrain patients or hold image receptors during exposure *shall* be provided with shielding, *e.g.*, leaded aprons, gloves.

3.1.4.2 *Extraoral Radiography.* Regulations, recommendations and procedures (NCRP, 1989a) from medical radiology, including positive beam-receptor alignment and collimation of the beam to the area of clinical interest, apply to extraoral dental projections. A few of these projections are peculiar to dental radiology. High-speed screen-film systems or digital image receptors meet the requirements of spatial and contrast resolution for these images.

The fastest imaging system consistent with the imaging task *shall* be used for all extraoral dental radiographic projections. High-speed (400 or greater) rare earth screen-film systems or digital-imaging systems of equivalent or greater speed *shall* be used.

Some digital-imaging systems are slower than the recommended 400 regular speed. These slower systems are not recommended for routine use.

3.1.4.2.1 *Panoramic radiography.* Panoramic images provide curved-plane tomograms of the teeth and jaws. The method is widely used in dental practice (Bohay *et al.*, 1995a; 1995b; 1998; Callen, 1994; Friedland, 1998; Kogon *et al.*, 1995). The major advantages are rapid acquisition of a single image encompassing the entire dental arches and their supporting structures, without the possibility of occasional discomfort of intraoral image receptor placement and minimal problems of infection control. Effective dose to the patient for a single panoramic image is approximately equal to that from four intraoral images, both using state-of-the-art technique (Gibbs, 2000). However, there are significant disadvantages that have radiation protection implications and need to be recognized by the dentist. Vertical image magnification is independent of horizontal magnification. The degree of magnification varies with position in the dental arch. This image distortion varies with anatomic area in a given patient and from patient to patient using the same panoramic x-ray machine. Further, repeat images of the same patient may show differing distortion because of slight differences in patient positioning. Image resolution is limited by the imperfect movement of source and image receptor required for the tomographic technique. Resolution is poorer than the dentist is accustomed to seeing from intraoral images and is likely to be inadequate for definitive diagnosis of incipient caries, beginning periapical lesions, or marginal periodontal disease (Flint *et al.*, 1998; Rumberg *et al.*, 1996).

The zone of sharp focus is limited and varies with manufacturer and model. It typically is designed to accommodate average adults; a few machines allow adjustment to patient dimensions. Patient positioning is critical and varies with manufacturer and model. Some use biteblocks that, if reusable, may present problems of infection control. Some machines allow only limited adjustment of beam parameters for factors such as image receptor speed and patient thickness. Older machines were designed for use with medium-speed calcium tungstate screen-film systems. In some cases the required reduction in x-ray output for use with high-speed rare-earth screen-film systems may be accomplished only by electronic modifications (prohibited by the federal performance standard) or by addition of filtration. Added filtration, unless compensated by lower kVp, hardens the beam spectrum, resulting in decreased image contrast. The dentist needs to be aware of these limitations in selecting and maintaining panoramic equipment or prescribing panoramic examinations. Otherwise, the limited diagnostic information obtained from the panoramic image may necessitate additional imaging. Periapical views alone may be adequate.

Panoramic x-ray machines *shall* be capable of operating at exposures appropriate for high-speed (400 or greater) rare-earth screen-film systems or digital image receptors of equivalent or greater speed.

3.1.4.2.2 *Cephalometric radiography.* The cephalometric technique provides reproducible radiographs of the facial structures. The principal application is evaluation of growth and development, as for orthodontic treatment. The equipment provides for positioning (and repositioning) of the patient together with alignment of beam, subject and image receptor. The source-to-skin distance is typically 150 cm or more, providing minimal geometric distortion in the image. It is frequently useful for the cephalometric image to show bony anatomy of the cranial base and facial skeleton plus the soft-tissue outline of facial contours, requiring image receptors of wide latitude. Filters that reduce exposure to the soft tissues of the facial profile have been used for this purpose (Freedman and Matteson, 1976). In some circumstances these filters have been placed at the image receptor instead of at the x-ray source.

Only the fastest screen-film system compatible with imaging requirements *shall* be used for the cephalometric image. Filters for imaging the soft tissues of the facial profile together with the facial skeleton *shall* be placed at the x-ray source rather than at the image receptor.

The cephalometric x-ray beam can be collimated to the area of clinical interest, which is almost always smaller than the dimensions of the image receptor. Cephalometric analysis of the usual lateral image does not require visualization of the dome of the calvarium or any structures posterior to the occipital condyles or inferior to the hyoid. Posterior-anterior cephalometric projections are also used; they also need not record structures superior to the cranial base or inferior to the hyoid. Practitioners need to remember that all structures recorded on the image need to be interpreted for evidence of disease or injury as well as for cephalometric analysis.

The x-ray beam for cephalometric radiography *shall* be collimated to the area of clinical interest.

3.1.4.3 *Fluoroscopy.* Real-time imaging, or fluoroscopy, is useful only for imaging changes in structures. Its use should be limited to those tasks requiring real-time imaging, such as the evaluation of moving anatomic structures (such as the temporomandibular joint) or the injection of radiographic contrast fluids (such as for sialography or temporomandibular joint arthrography). Fluoroscopy requires electronic image intensification and video display to minimize patient exposure; this equipment is expensive and not usually found in dental facilities. Further, dental x-ray machines are not generally capable of providing the required continuous radiation exposure.

Fluoroscopy *shall not* be used for static imaging in dental radiography.

3.1.5 *Film Processing*

Maintenance of image quality and minimum patient exposure depend on proper film processing. Film manufacturers prescribe or recommend processing chemicals and procedures matched to the film emulsion. Like all chemical processes, the time required for image development to progress to completion is inversely proportional to temperature. Therefore, development time is adjusted for the temperature of the solution. This time-temperature method of ensuring complete development may be achieved by either manual or automatic processing. When development is incomplete, x-ray exposure is increased to provide useful image density. The combination of increased exposure and incomplete development results in not only needless overexposure of the patient but also decreased image contrast.

Dental radiographic films *shall* be developed according to the film manufacturer's instructions, using the time-temperature method and recommended chemistry or its equivalent. Sight developing *shall not* be used.

3.1.6 *Digital Image Postprocessing*

A major advantage of digital imaging is the ability to alter image properties after acquisition. It is possible to make certain features more obvious by procedures such as adjustment of image density and contrast (technically called window level and width); or image reversal, or exchange of the "negative" radiographic image for a "positive" like a photographic print. These procedures may compensate for over- or underexposure, eliminating the need for retake of a poorly exposed image. However, these procedures allow the injudicious use of routine over- or underexposure, each with undesirable consequences. Overexposures needlessly increase patient dose without significant benefit. Underexposure results in decreased signal-to-noise ratio (Appendix E), resulting in loss of diagnostic information as the image becomes "grainy" or "snowy." Further, uninformed or injudicious use of these procedures may produce the appearance of disease where it does not exist (false positive) or absence of disease where it exists (false negative) (Tsang *et al.*, 1999).

Radiographic techniques for digital imaging *shall* be adjusted for the minimum patient dose required to produce a signal-to-noise ratio sufficient to provide image quality to meet the purpose of the examination.

3.1.7 *Interpretation*

Unnecessary exposure in radiography may be due to inadequate evaluation and interpretation, resulting in diagnostic errors and unproductive radiation exposure. For maximum diagnostic yield at minimum exposure, image evaluation and interpretation is best carried out in a quiet atmosphere, free from distractions (Wuehrmann, 1970). Perception of image details has been shown to be maximum when the illuminated surface of the view box not covered with films and opaque film mounts is masked with opaque material to eliminate glare, variable luminance of the view-box lamp is available, room illumination is reduced to the level of the displayed films, and a magnifier is used.

3.1.8 *Leaded Aprons*

Leaded aprons for patients were first recommended in dentistry many years ago when dental x-ray equipment was much less sophisticated and films much slower than current standards. They provided a quick fix for the poorly collimated and unfiltered dental x-ray beams of the era. Gonadal (or whole-body) doses from these early full-mouth examinations, reported as large as 50 mGy (Budowsky *et al.*, 1956), could be reduced substantially by leaded aprons. Gonadal doses from current panoramic or full-mouth intraoral examinations using state-of-the-art technology and procedures do not exceed 5 μGy (5×10^{-3} mGy) (White, 1992). A significant portion of this gonadal dose results from scattered radiation arising within the patient's body. Leaded aprons do not significantly reduce these doses. Technological and procedural improvements have eliminated the requirement for the leaded apron, provided all other recommendations of this Report are rigorously followed (NRPB, 2001). However, some patients have come to expect the apron and may request that it be used. Its use remains a prudent but not essential practice.

The use of leaded aprons on patients *shall not* be required if all other recommendations in this Report are rigorously followed. However, if under exceptional circumstances any of these recommendations are not implemented in a specific case, then the leaded apron *should* be used.

3.1.9 *Thyroid Collars*

The thyroid gland, especially in children, is among the most sensitive organs to radiation-induced tumors, both benign and malignant (Appendix B). Even with optimum techniques, the primary dental x-ray beam may still pass near and occasionally through the gland. If the x-ray beam is properly collimated to the size of the image receptor or area of clinical interest, and exposure of the gland is still unavoidable, any attempt to shield the gland would interfere with the production of a clinically-useful image. However, in those occasional uncooperative patients for whom rectangular collimation and positive beam-receptor alignment cannot be achieved for intraoral radiographs, then thyroid shielding may reduce dose to the gland without interfering with image production (NRPB, 2001).

Thyroid shielding *shall* be provided for children, and *should* be provided for adults, when it will not interfere with the examination.

3.2 Protection of the Operator

Equipment and procedures that reduce patient exposure will also reduce exposure of the operator and the environment. Additional measures, however, will further reduce occupational and public exposure without affecting patient dose or image quality.

3.2.1 *Shielding Design*

Attention to office layout and shielding design provide convenient methods for implementing the ALARA principle. Shielding does not necessarily mean lead-lined x-ray rooms. Normal building materials may be sufficient in most cases. Expert guidance can provide effective shielding design at nominal incremental cost (Appendix F), with protection by barriers, distance from x-ray source, and operator position.

> **Shielding design by a qualified expert *shall* be provided for all new or remodeled dental facilities. When a conventional building structure does not provide adequate shielding, the shielding *shall* be increased by providing greater thickness of building materials or by adding lead, gypsum wallboard, concrete, steel or other suitable material. Adequacy of shielding *shall* be determined by calculation and checked by survey measurements.**

It is in the economic best interest of the dentist to obtain shielding design by a qualified expert at the design stage. For a new or remodeled facility, proper shielding design can usually provide radiation protection to meet shielding design goals (Appendix F) at little or no incremental construction cost. However, if measurements after construction is finished indicate that these requirements are not met, the cost of retrofitting might be considerable.

Several commercial and noncommercial software packages are available to perform shielding calculations. Such software may be employed only if the user is fully aware of its underlying assumptions and limitations. In particular, the leakage radiation characteristics of dental x-ray housings may be significantly different from that of medical diagnostic x-ray housings. Uninformed use of software cannot be substituted for consultation with a qualified expert.

3.2.1.1 *Barriers.* It is a fundamental principle of radiation protection that no one other than the patient undergoing the procedure is permitted in the room at the time of radiation exposure. Fixed barriers, generally walls, provide the most economical, effective and convenient means of excluding office staff from the primary x-ray beam as it exits the patient or from radiation scattered from the patient or other objects in the primary beam.

Shielding design for new offices *shall* provide protective barriers for the operator. The barriers *shall* be constructed so operators can maintain visual contact and communication with patients throughout the procedures.

3.2.1.2 *Distance*. In some existing facilities, design precludes use of a protective barrier.

In the absence of a barrier in an existing facility, the operator *shall* remain at least 2 m from the tube head during exposure. If the 2 m distance cannot be maintained, then a barrier *shall* be provided.

3.2.1.3 *Position*. If the facility design requires that the operator be in the room at the time of exposure, then the operator should be positioned not only at maximum distance (at least 2 m) from the tube head, but also at the location of minimum exposure (Figure 3.3). Maximum exposure will generally be in the primary beam as it exits the patient. Maximum scattered radiation will be backwards, *i.e.*, 90 to 180 degrees from the primary beam as it enters the patient. Generally the position of minimum exposure will be at 45 degrees from the primary beam as it exits the patient (de Haan and van Aken, 1990).

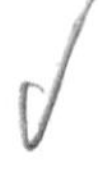

3.2.2 *Personal Dosimeters*

Monitoring of individual occupational exposures is generally required if it can be reasonably expected that any dental staff member will receive a significant dose. NCRP (1998) recommends provision of monitors to all personnel who are likely to receive an effective dose greater than 1 mSv y^{-1}. It needs to be emphasized that this recommendation concerns effective dose, which is generally much less than monitor readings (Appendix C). The most recent available data (Table 2.1) indicate that the average annual occupational dose in dentistry in the United States in 1980 was 0.2 mSv (Kumazawa *et al.*, 1984). Few dental workers received more than 1 mSv and 68 percent received exposures below the threshold of detection.

World data for the period 1990 to 1994 show a mean annual occupational dose of 0.06 mSv for dental workers (UNSCEAR, 2000). These data suggest that dental personnel are not expected to receive occupational exposures greater than the recommended threshold for monitoring of 1 mSv y^{-1}. However, the limit applicable

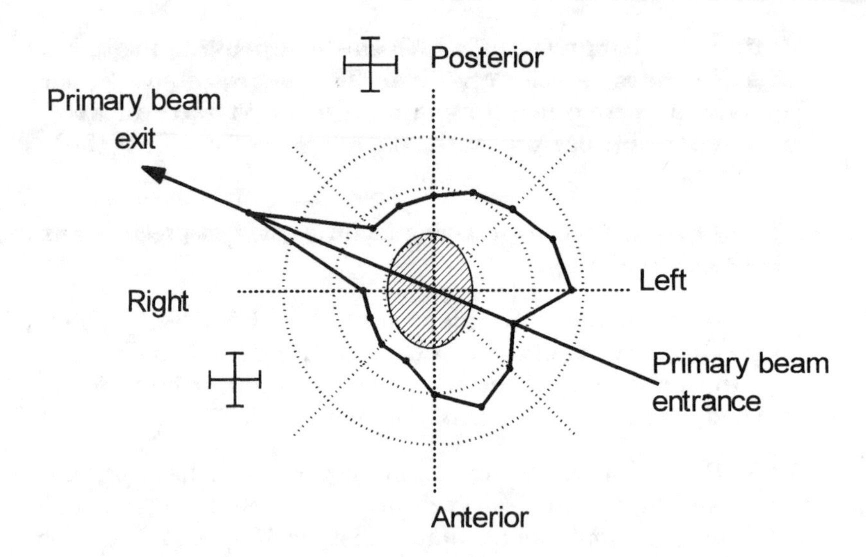

Fig. 3.3. Operator exposure as a function of position in room relative to patient and primary beam. View from above for a left molar bitewing. The heavy line in the polar coordinate plot indicates dose by its distance from the center of the plot. Maximum dose is in the exit beam. The recommended positions for minimum exposures (crosses) are at 45 degrees from the exit beam. Note that most scattered radiation is backward (de Haan and van Aken, 1990).

to pregnant workers of 0.5 mSv equivalent dose to the fetus per month once pregnancy is known, suggest that personal dosimetry may be a prudent practice for those workers. Current regulations require that dosimeters be obtained from services accredited for accuracy and reproducibility. These services distribute dosimeter packets regularly; the facility returns the packets to the service after use (generally monthly or quarterly) for readout and report.

Provision of personal dosimeters for external exposure measurement *should* be considered for workers who are likely to receive an annual effective dose in excess of 1 mSv.

Personal dosimeters *shall* be provided for known pregnant occupationally-exposed personnel.

3.3 Protection of the Public

For shielding design purposes, the public includes all individuals who are in uncontrolled areas such as reception rooms, other treatment rooms or in adjacent corridors in the building within or outside of the dental facility (NCRP, 2000; in press). The popular "open design" dental facility, which places two or more treatment chairs in a single room, may present problems.

A patient in the room during diagnostic exposure of another patient *shall* be treated as a member of the public. When portable x-ray machines are used, all individuals in the environs (*e.g.*, other patients, their families, etc.) *shall* be protected as members of the public.

Based on NCRP (1993a) and the International Commission on Radiological Protection (ICRP, 1991) recommendations for the annual limit on effective dose to a member of the general public, shielding designs need to limit exposure to all individuals in uncontrolled areas to an effective dose that does not exceed 1 mSv y^{-1}. After a review of the application of the guidance in NCRP (1993a) to medical (and dental) facilities, NCRP has concluded that a suitable source constraint for shielding individual members of the public in or near such facilities is an effective dose of 1 mSv in any year (NCRP, in press). This recommendation can be achieved with a weekly shielding design goal of 0.02 mGy air kerma (*i.e.*, an annual air-kerma value of 1 mGy for uncontrolled areas) (Appendix F).

New dental facilities *shall* be designed such that no individual member of the public will receive an effective dose in excess of 1 mSv annually.

3.4 Quality Assurance

Radiation exposure to patient, operator and the public can be reduced by minimizing the need for repeat exposures because of inadequate image quality (NRPB, 2001). The term "quality assurance" describes a program for periodic assessment of the performance of all parts of the radiologic procedure (NCRP, 1988; Valachovic *et al.*, 1981). In addition to determination of x-ray machine performance by a qualified expert (Appendix C), film processing chemistry and procedures, image receptor performance characteristics, and darkroom integrity need to be evaluated at appropriate intervals (AADR, 1983; NCHCT, 1981; Valachovic *et al.*, 1981). These routine quality-assurance procedures can be performed by properly-trained dental office staff.

A written protocol for periodic quality assurance *shall* be developed and implemented for each x-ray machine, image receptor system, and processor or darkroom.

3.4.1 *Equipment Performance*

Dental x-ray machines are inspected at regular intervals to ensure that they are functioning within specifications. These inspections are performed by a qualified expert.

All new dental x-ray installations and existing installations not previously surveyed *shall* have a radiation protection survey performed by, or under the direction of, a qualified expert. Resurveys *shall* be performed at regular intervals thereafter. The resurvey interval *should not* exceed 4 y. In addition, a resurvey *shall* be made after any change in the installation, workload, or operating conditions that might significantly increase occupational or public exposure (including x-ray machine service or repair that could affect the x-ray machine output or performance).

3.4.2 *Film Processing*

Darkroom solutions are subject to gradual deterioration. The deterioration may go unnoticed as it becomes severe enough to degrade image quality. Daily determinations are required to prevent this degradation in a typical dental facility.

Darkroom chemistry and each film processor used in the facility *shall* be evaluated daily for performance, *i.e.*, constancy of optical density and contrast, and overall quality of the resulting films.

3.4.2.1 *Sensitometry and Densitometry.* The most sensitive and rigorous method of darkroom quality assurance requires the use of a sensitometer, a precise optical device to expose a film to produce a defined pattern of optical densities in the processed film. These densities are then measured with a densitometer, and compared to the densities in a similarly-exposed film previously processed in fresh solutions under ideal conditions. A daily log is maintained; any change indicates a problem with processing, either development time or temperature or contaminated solutions. This method requires additional equipment but only a few minutes of operator time to execute. It is highly recommended for the busy facility, but simpler, less costly methods may be adequate for average dental offices.

3.4.2.2 *Stepwedge.* A standard radiographic film exposed through an aluminum stepwedge (Figure 3.4) to a defined x-ray exposure may be substituted for the sensitometrically-exposed film. The stepwedge may be purchased at nominal cost, fabricated by a machine shop, or fabricated in the office using lead foil backings from dental film packets (Valachovic *et al.*, 1981). Overall size of the stepwedge should be similar to that of a standard intraoral film. It is made to resemble stairs. Each step of an aluminum stepwedge is 1 mm thick and about 3 to 4 mm wide. There should be at least six steps. Exposure parameters, including x-ray machine settings and exposure geometry are reproduced precisely for each exposure. The structure on which the film is placed will provide backscattered radiation that will affect film density. Thus the film and source are placed in the same position on the same structure for each exposure. The processed film is then compared visually with a reference film identically exposed and processed in fresh

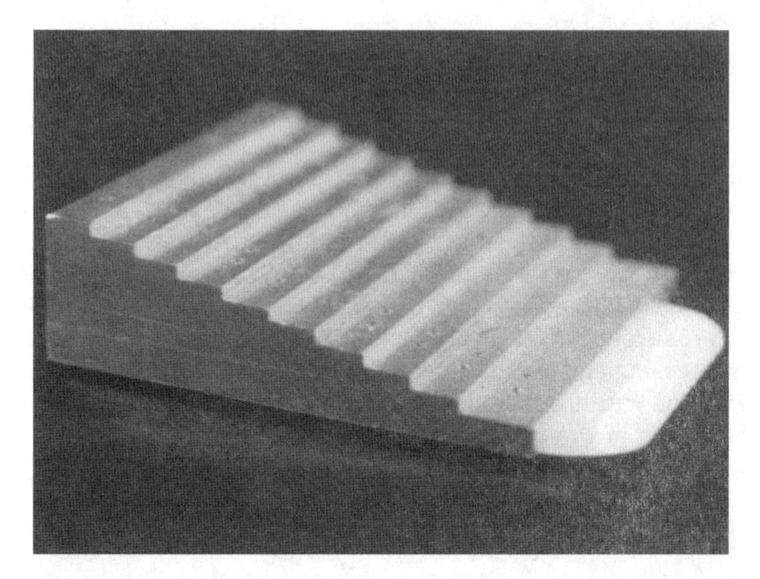

Fig. 3.4. Machined aluminum stepwedge, placed over an intraoral film packet. Each step is 1 mm in depth and 3 mm wide. An effective stepwedge can be constructed from a stack of layers of aluminum or lead foil. It is used for exposing test films for quality assurance.

solutions under ideal conditions. Devices that facilitate this process are commercially available at modest cost. A reproducible change of one step or more in density, which is readily detectable visually and readily confirmed by repeating the test, should signal the need for corrective action. The change in density may be the result of either a different x-ray exposure or differences in processing. Darkroom problems are more likely and should be corrected first. This method is less sensitive than sensitometry and densitometry but should suffice for many dental facilities.

3.4.2.3 *Reference Film*. Use of a properly exposed and processed intraoral film as a reference has been proposed as another method of quality assurance (AADR, 1983; Valachovic *et al.*, 1981). When using this method, a high-quality film is attached to a corner of the view box. Subsequent clinical films can then be compared with this reference film. This method is not as sensitive or reliable as a sensitometry and densitometry or a stepwedge, and is not recommended for routine use. In rare circumstances it may be used as a stopgap measure, usually in facilities with very low radiographic workload (fewer than 10 intraoral films per week).

3.4.3 *Image Receptor*

Radiographic films, screen-film systems, and digital image receptors constitute an important part of radiology. Their performance is tested periodically to ensure that they function according to specifications.

3.4.3.1 *Film*. Unexposed film may become "fogged" by gradual chemical deterioration, which is temperature dependent and therefore may be slowed by storing film in a refrigerator. Alternatively, stray light or x rays may produce an increase in density of exposed or unexposed film. Exposure to certain chemicals, heat or pressure may produce fog or other artifacts. These artifacts may be detected by processing and evaluating an unexposed film. Evaluation is best performed with a densitometer but may be approximated by visual comparison of the current film with an unfogged film from a new box and processed in fresh solutions.

Each type of film used in the facility *shall* be evaluated for fog and artifacts monthly and each time a new box or batch of film is opened. When excessive fog is identified, the affected box or batch of film *shall* be discarded or returned to the vendor for replacement.

3.4.3.2 *Screen-Film Systems.* Both cassettes and screens may acquire defects during normal use. Integrity of cassettes is determined by visual inspection and by processing of an unexposed film that has been in the cassette for at least 1 h while the cassette is exposed to normal room illumination. Light leaks from the cassette will appear as dark streaks on the film. Screens are evaluated visually for surface defects such as scratches or fingerprints. Screen maintenance requires periodic cleaning, following the manufacturer's instructions. Poor screen-film contact leads to unsharpness in images. Screen-film contact and uniformity of response are best evaluated by exposing a film (in its cassette) overlaid with a piece of copper test screen. Visual inspection of the processed film for sharpness and uniformity of the image can assess performance of the imaging system.

Screen-film cassettes, including screens, *shall* be visually evaluated after any accident (such as dropping) for integrity and performance. Tests for screen-film contact *should* be performed every six months. Any defective items *shall* be promptly repaired or replaced.

3.4.3.3 *Digital-Imaging Systems.* Procedures for evaluating the performance of digital-imaging systems are quite different from those used with film or screen-film image receptors. By using appropriately designed phantoms and software, image quality aspects such as resolution, contrast, signal-to-noise ratio, and contrast-to-noise ratio may be measured directly. However, the required standards, apparatus and software for dental systems do not currently exist. These limitations are important factors when considering the purchase of digital-imaging systems.

3.4.4 *Darkroom Integrity*

Each darkroom is evaluated for light leaks and safelight performance. A "coin test" is performed by placing an unexposed unwrapped intraoral film at a normal working position and putting a coin upon it. After a time equivalent to a normal darkroom procedure (such as processing films from a typical clinical procedure), the film is processed. An image of the coin indicates a problem with either light leaks or the safelight. Repeating the procedure with the safelight off will determine which was the source of the problem. These tests are performed monthly or following a change in safelight filter or lamp. Direct exposure films have different spectral sensitivities from those used with screens; a safelight filter appropriate for one may not be adequate for the other.

Daylight loaders are commonly used with automatic dental film processors, eliminating the need for the darkroom. These systems provide light-tight boxes attached to the processor loading areas. Each box contains a port for placing exposed films (still in their wrappers or cassettes) in the box, ports for inserting the hands so the operator may manipulate films in the box, and a viewing port with a filter similar to the safelight filter. The safelight filter is designed for use in a darkroom with low-level illumination; it may not provide adequate protection for a daylight loader used in a normally-illuminated room. It may be necessary to use daylight loaders only in rooms with reduced illumination. Further, the daylight loader may present difficulties in infection control with intraoral film wrappers contaminated with oral fluids. Like the darkroom, the daylight loader may be evaluated for light leaks using the "coin test."

Each darkroom and daylight loader *shall* be evaluated for integrity at initial installation, and then monthly and following change of room lighting or darkroom safelight lamp or filter.

3.4.5 *Leaded Aprons and Thyroid Collars*

Minimum acceptable evaluation of leaded aprons and thyroid collars consists of periodic visual inspection for defects. More functional evaluation, when available, consists of fluoroscopy to detect hidden shielding defects.

Leaded aprons and thyroid collars *shall* be visually inspected for defects at monthly intervals or more frequently if they are damaged. Fluoroscopic examination for hidden defects *should* be performed annually.

3.4.6 *Documentation*

It is essential that all quality-assurance procedures, together with their results and any corrective actions, be documented. This information is critical in troubleshooting chronic problems. Comparison of new results with previous ones may be the best way to detect any change in performance of equipment or procedures.

A log of all quality-assurance procedures *shall* be maintained. The log *shall* contain date, procedure, results, and any corrective action.

3.4.7 *Suggested Quality-Assurance Procedures*

The following outline of a recommended basic quality-assurance protocol for a typical private dental office is given in Valachovic *et al.* (1981):

Daily
- replenish processing solutions
- check temperature of processing solutions
- perform sensitometry and densitometry, or stepwedge test
- enter findings in quality-assurance log

Weekly
- clean processing equipment
- evaluate processing solutions and replace, if necessary
- check and clean view boxes
- document in quality-assurance log
- review quality-assurance log and adequacy of corrective actions

Monthly
- check darkroom and safelight for leaks using coin test
- check and clean all intensifying screens
- check that exposure charts are posted at each x-ray machine
- inspect leaded aprons and thyroid collars

Yearly to quadrennially
- calibrate all x-ray machines (Appendix C)

Some authorities have recommended or prescribed quality-assurance procedures including other issues. Some of these reflect differences between nations or legal jurisdictions in legal requirements. For example, in the United Kingdom, quality assurance also involves frequent evaluations of image quality, as well as working procedures, training and audits (NRPB, 2001). Further, all retakes are required to be justified and recorded.

3.5 Training

NCRP Reports No. 127 and No. 134 (NCRP, 1998; 2000) recommend that all dental personnel be appropriately trained in radiation protection. Basic familiarity with radiation protection can be expected in those who by education and certification are credentialed to expose radiographs [*i.e.*, dentists, registered dental hygienists, certified dental assistants, and radiographic (or dental radiographic) technologists]. Curricula for their education are subject to recommendations by various professional organizations and requirements of accrediting and credentialing agencies. In the United Kingdom, the National Radiological Protection Board provided specific recommendations for education of dentists in radiology, including radiation protection (NRPB, 1994). These recommendations included credentialing of faculty and adequacy of resources and curriculum for undergraduate education, and required frequency of continuing education. Others have shown that dentists who are better informed in radiation science are more likely to adopt modern dose-sparing technology (Svenson *et al.*, 1997b; 1998).

Accrediting agencies *should* re-evaluate the adequacy of their criteria for undergraduate education of dentists and auxiliaries, together with implementation of the criteria in educational institutions.

The ability of office personnel to understand and implement all of the recommendations in this Report cannot be assumed. Other personnel (*e.g.*, secretaries, receptionists, laboratory technologists) who are not credentialed for performing radiographic procedures may be subjected to incidental contact with radiation. These personnel are likely to have received little or no training or experience in radiation protection.

The dentist or other designated individual *shall* provide training in radiation protection for all dental personnel sufficient to ensure that they understand and comply with all recommendations in this Report.

Opportunities *should* be provided for auxiliary personnel to attend appropriate continuing education courses.

The required training may be provided by any combination of self-instruction (including reading), group instruction, mentoring, or on-the-job training. Periodic evaluation of staff practices will determine the need, if any, for retraining. Essential topics to be covered in the training program include:

- risks related to exposure to radiation and to other hazards in the workplace
- dose limits
- sources of exposure
- basic protective measures
- security
- warning signs, postings, labeling and alarms
- responsibility of each person
- overall safety in the workplace
- specific facility hazards
- special requirements for women of reproductive age
- regulatory and licensure requirements
- infection control
- the ALARA principle

This training may be expedited by the development and maintenance of a site-specific radiation protection manual.

The technology of dental radiology is changing rapidly. Continuing education resources are generally available to keep the dentist apprised of new developments.

The dentist *should* regularly attend continuing education courses in all aspects of dental radiology, including radiation protection.

3.6 Infection Control

Dental radiologic procedures are conducted using universal precautions that prevent transfer of infectious agents among patients, operator and office staff. All equipment and procedures need to be compatible with current infection control philosophy and techniques, while still maintaining the ALARA principle. It is important that a rigorous, written infection control policy (Appendix A) be developed and routinely applied. These practices apply especially to intraoral radiography, in which multiple projections are commonly used in a single examination. The image receptors are placed in a contaminated environment. Gloved hands of the operator who is observing universal precautions can become contaminated when placing image receptors in the mouth or removing exposed ones from the mouth. This contamination then can be easily spread, such as to the x-ray machine and to image processing equipment. Universal precautions are measures mandated by the Occupational Safety and Health Administration to prevent dissemination of contamination (Appendix A).

4. Role of Equipment Design

Optimum use of x rays in dental diagnosis and treatment (*i.e.*, maximum information at minimum exposure of patient, operator and the public) requires adherence of equipment to certain fundamental design principles. The Food and Drug Administration (FDA) has developed performance standards for medical and dental x-ray machines. Compliance with these standards at installation is required of all medical and dental x-ray machines manufactured since 1974 in the United States (FDA, 1995). Compliance with international standards is also recommended (IEC, 1994).

Dental x-ray machines *shall* comply with all applicable laws, standards and regulations governing their manufacture, installation and use, and with all recommendations in this Report. Older equipment *shall* be brought into compliance with these requirements and recommendations or be replaced.

The peculiarities of dental radiology impose requirements in addition to those of the FDA performance standard. Design of x-ray equipment in accord with these requirements and recommendations includes provision for users to apply modern clinical techniques.

4.1 Image Receptors

The fastest available image receptors are specified in this Report for all dental radiological procedures (Appendix E). Users are required to update their techniques as faster image receptors become available. It is incumbent on manufacturers to enable users to meet these requirements.

Dental x-ray machines *shall* provide a range of exposures suitable for use with the fastest image receptors appropriate for those clinical procedures for

which the machine was designed and available at the time of machine manufacture. To avoid rapid obsolescence, this range *should* include exposures for image receptors of at least twice the speed of techniques at that time.

4.2 Intraoral Radiography

Additional requirements are imposed on x-ray machines designed for use with intraoral image receptors.

4.2.1 *Tube Head Stability*

The articulated arm that supports the tube head or diagnostic source assembly needs to be capable of achieving any position and angulation required for intraoral radiography, and maintaining it until the exposure is complete.

The tube head *shall* achieve a stable position, free of drift and oscillation, within 1 s after its release at the desired operating position. Drift during that 1 s *shall* be no greater than 0.5 cm. The operator *shall not* hold the tube head during exposure.

4.2.2 *Collimation*

Requirements for beam collimation for intraoral imaging in this Report are more rigorous than many previously published (Section 3.1.4.1.3). Equipment design needs to provide for these more restrictive techniques.

Equipment designed for use with intraoral image receptors *shall* be capable of providing rectangular collimation to approximate the dimensions of the image receptor. The linear dimensions of the beam in each axis *should not* exceed those of the receptor by more than two percent of the source-to-image receptor distance. This collimation may be inherent in the x-ray machine position-indicating device or may be accomplished by accessory devices.

4.3 Panoramic Radiography

The rotational panoramic tomographic technique uses a narrow vertical beam, exposing only a small portion of the image receptor at any one time. The image receptor shifts during panoramic motion, resulting in exposure of the entire receptor. Panoramic x-ray beams must be no larger than the area of receptor exposed to the beam at any point in time. This area is defined by the slit collimator at the tube head.

The x-ray beam for rotational panoramic tomography *shall* be collimated such that its vertical dimension is no greater than that required to expose the area of clinical interest. In no case *shall* it be larger than the slit in the image-receptor carrier plus a tolerance of two percent of the source-to-image receptor distance.

4.4 Cephalometric Radiography

The area of clinical interest in cephalometric radiography is usually significantly smaller than the image receptor. Thus, collimation to the size of the image receptor does not meet the intent of restricting the beam to image only those structures of clinical interest (Section 3.1.4.2.2). The central axis of the beam is usually aligned through external auditory canals, which are positioned by the ear rods of the cephalostat. Imaging of structures superior to the superior orbital rim, posterior to occipital condyles, and inferior to the hyoid bone is clinically unnecessary. The desired collimation is asymmetric, and the central axis of the beam is not centered on the image receptor. Further, it is usually desirable to image the soft-tissue facial profile along with the osseous structures of the face; this is accomplished by reducing exposure to the anterior soft tissues.

X-ray equipment for cephalometric radiography *shall* provide for asymmetric collimation of the beam to the area of clinical interest. The collimator *should* include a wedge filter to reduce exposure to the soft-tissue facial profile such that it may be imaged.

4.5 Multiple X-Ray Tube Installations

Modern equipment provides for operation of several x-ray tubes, in several rooms, from a single control panel. The tubes may include intraoral, panoramic and cephalometric.

In multiple x-ray tube installations, there *shall* be indication at the tube when it is connected and ready for use, and at the control panel of which tube is connected. It *shall not* be possible to energize more than one tube at a time. The patient at any tube *shall* be visible to the operator during exposure.

The control panel *shall* indicate when x rays are being generated and which x-ray tube is energized. The operating potential (kVp), x-ray tube current (if variable) and exposure time *shall* be indicated.

5. Role of the Qualified Expert

A qualified (and credentialed) expert should serve as a consultant to the dentist in designing, implementing and maintaining radiation protection programs, particularly with regard to shielding design (Appendix F) and equipment surveys (Appendix C).

5.1 Shielding Design

Shielding design is included in facility planning (before floor plans are completed) to ensure that neither occupational nor public doses exceed recommended limits. The qualified expert may present more than one shielding design for a facility. Each design may include office layouts, equipment locations, doorway positions, construction of partitions, etc. Construction costs for each design generally (but not always) vary directly with the magnitude of dose reduction. With innovative design, dose reductions can be achieved at little or no cost and without adverse impact on patient care (*i.e.*, the ALARA principle).

5.2 Equipment Surveys

Surveys of x-ray equipment are performed to determine compliance with laws and regulations governing the use of that equipment and to ensure that the equipment is being used in a manner compatible with standards of good radiologic practice (NRPB, 2001). Newly-installed equipment also needs to comply with the federal performance standard (FDA, 1995); this compliance is certified by the equipment installer. However, performance of new equipment is determined by the qualified expert. Any deviations are reported to the dentist, who is responsible for corrective action. The qualified expert should also report to the dentist any operational changes that may improve radiation protection programs.

6. Conclusions

Dentists who conduct their radiology practices in accordance with the requirements and suggestions in this Report can obtain maximum benefit to the oral health of their patients and minimum radiation exposure to patient, operator and the public. All of the factors addressed in this Report are important and interrelated. Quality practice dictates that none be neglected. The technical factors, including office design and shielding, equipment design, clinical techniques, image receptors, darkroom procedures, and quality assurance are essential. However, the professional skill and judgment of the dentist in prescribing radiologic examinations and interpreting the results are paramount.

There is no conclusive proof that the radiation exposure from dental x rays is harmful. A few epidemiological studies have demonstrated statistically-significant associations between dental x-ray exposure and cancer (*e.g.*, Graham *et al.*, 1966; Preston-Martin *et al.*, 1988). These studies do not demonstrate cause-and-effect. If a substantial risk existed, it would have been identified and reported. It seems reasonable to conclude that radiation-related risks to dental patients and dental x-ray equipment operators are numerically very small and may be zero.

Patient doses from dental radiographic procedures are low (Tables 6.1 and 6.2), especially in comparison with those from many medical radiologic procedures (Table 6.2) and environmental exposure (Figure 2.1). White (1992) has surveyed available data and concluded that the values for dental x-ray exposures in the tables are representative. More recent studies have substantiated these conclusions (Avendanio *et al.*, 1996; Cederburg *et al.*, 1997; Williams and Montgomery, 2000). The United Nations Scientific Committee on the Effects of Atomic Radiation (UNSCEAR, 2000) presented average effective doses of 1.3×10^{-2} mSv per intraoral examination (type and number of images not specified) and 1.2×10^{-2} mSv per panoramic examination. These doses are much smaller than the minimum doses for which coefficients of risk per unit dose can be meaningfully applied (NCRP, 1993b). They are numerically equal to the unavoidable natural environmental exposure received in a few hours to a few days by the average American.

TABLE 6.1—*Patient radiation doses from intraoral dental radiography.*

kVp	Cone	Beam	Geometry	Effective Dose (in μSv) per Examination[a]			
				FMX[b]		BWX[c]	
				Film Speed[d]		Film Speed[d]	
				D	E	D	E
70	Long[e]	Rectangular	Parallel	29	15	5	3
	Long	Round	Parallel	150	76	23	12
	Short[f]	Round	Bisect angle	200	100	27	14
80	Long	Rectangular	Parallel	26	13	5	3
	Long	Round	Parallel	130	67	20	11
	Short	Round	Bisect angle	170	87	23	13
90	Long	Rectangular	Parallel	25	14	5	3
	Long	Round	Parallel	120	68	20	11
	Short	Round	Bisect angle	150	85	22	12

[a]Recalculated from data of Gibbs *et al*. (1988a). 1,000 μSv = 1 mSv (*e.g.*, 150 μSv = 0.15 mSv).
[b]FMX, full-mouth series of periapical views, usually 14 to 21 films. May also include bitewing projections.
[c]BWX, examination consisting of bitewing projections, usually only of posterior teeth. Generally two or four films.
[d]See Glossary for explanation of film speed.
[e]Source-to-image receptor distance, 40 cm.
[f]Source-to-image receptor distance, 20 cm.

TABLE 6.2—*Patient doses from diagnostic examinations.*

Examination[a]	Effective Dose (in mSv) per Examination
Dental panoramic[b]	6×10^{-3} to 1.1×10^{-2}
Cephalometric[c]	1.7×10^{-2}
TMJ tomogram[c,d]	2×10^{-3}
Chest (posteroanterior and lateral)[e]	0.17
Chest[f]	4×10^{-2}
CT chest[f]	7.8
Skull[f]	0.10
CT head[f]	1.8
Abdomen[f]	1.2
CT abdomen[f]	7.6
Thoracic spine[f]	1.0
Lumbar spine[f]	2.1
Pelvis[f]	1.1
CT pelvis[f]	7.1
IVP[f]	4.2
Barium enema[f]	8.7
Mammography[f]	1×10^{-2}

[a]CT = computed tomography
IVP = intravenous pyelogram
TMJ = temporomandibular joint
[b]Recalculated from data of Gibbs *et al.* (1988b).
[c]Gibbs (2000).
[d]Conventional, per image.
[e]Recalculated from data of Gibbs (1989).
[f]Data from ICRP (1993).

There are no recent published data concerning the frequency of dental radiographic examinations in the United States. UNSCEAR (2000) presented data on frequency of medical and dental radiologic procedures in many nations. The data included medical examinations in the United States, but not dental. UNSCEAR (2000) reported an annual average of 365 intraoral and 41 panoramic examinations per 1,000 population in health care Level 1 (*i.e.*, developed) nations, mostly in western Europe, the Western Hemisphere, and the Middle East. Extrapolation of these data to the American population poses obvious problems.

Dental radiographic procedures are very common but the associated x-ray doses are quite low. Application of the ALARA principle to reduction of these doses is justified. For intraoral radiography, changing from D- to E- or F-speed film or to modern digital image receptors results in dose reduction by factors of at least two. Introduction of rectangular collimation to replace the 7 cm round beam reduces dose by factors of four to five. Both of these are accomplished at little or no cost, and together may result in tenfold reductions in effective doses.

Finally, the concept of informed consent requires that dental patients be provided with information as to the benefits and risks of dental procedures, including dental radiography. This Section provides the dentist with data (*e.g.*, Tables 6.1 and 6.2) on the magnitude of effective doses from typical dental x-ray procedures, and general statements are given in this Section that can be used to inform the patient about the radiation doses from dental x-ray procedures and the nature of risk associated with these doses. Additional background on radiation risk assessment is found in Appendix B. Dentists are encouraged to use this information to educate their patients as opportunity provides.

Appendix A

Radiography-Related Biohazards

Infection control influences all aspects of oral radiography. The risk of transmission of infectious disease in the x-ray operatory and darkroom impacts the dentist, staff and patients alike. Thus, effective infection control measures need to be included in the performance of oral radiographic procedures. This Appendix includes reference to selected Occupational Safety and Health Administration regulations (OSHA, 1994a; 1994b; 2001) that may apply to oral radiographic procedures.

A.1 Infection Control

A written infection control policy needs to be maintained that includes the performance of oral radiographic procedures (Brand *et al.*, 1992; CDC, 2003). The Centers for Disease Control and Prevention (CDC) recommend that all personnel who are subject to occupational exposure to blood-borne pathogens or other biological hazards receive infection-control training on initial assignment, plus retraining at least annually and when new tasks affect their occupational exposure (CDC, 2003; OSHA, 2001).

A.1.1 *Facilities and Equipment*

Surfaces that may become contaminated during oral radiographic procedures are covered with plastic wrap, aluminum foil, or moisture-proof paper that is changed between patients (ADA, 1996; CDC, 2003; OSHA, 2001). Items used in conjunction with direct digital radiography that may become contaminated and cannot be heat-sterilized, such as the x-ray sensor, connecting cord, and computer equipment, are covered with FDA-cleared protective barriers during patient treatment or imaging. Further, high-level disinfection is recommended between patients, using an U.S. Environmental Protection Agency (EPA) registered hospital disinfectant. The recommendations of the equipment manufacturer should be consulted for methods of disinfection and sterilization of digital radiographic apparatus.

Uncovered surfaces that become contaminated are cleaned and disinfected with an EPA-registered hospital-level disinfectant with low (human immunodificiency virus and hepatitis B virus label claims) to intermediate (tuberculocidal claim) activity after each patient (CDC, 2003; OSHA, 2001). If there is visible blood contamination, use an intermediate-level disinfectant. If sodium hypochlorite is chosen for disinfection, an EPA-registered product is preferable. If this is not available, a 1:100 dilution of household chlorine bleach is an inexpensive and effective alternative. Chlorine solutions are corrosive to metals, especially aluminum (ADA, 1996; CDC, 2003). Fixed items, such as ear rods, chin rests, and head positioners cannot be removed for sterilization and need to be covered or cleaned and disinfected with an appropriate EPA-registered surface disinfectant (or sodium hypochlorite) (Brand *et al.*, 1992).

Technologic advances to minimize contamination during oral radiographic procedures, such as foot controls for chair adjustment and x-ray exposure, are encouraged. Disposable items eliminate the need for sterilization between patients, and may be dispensed in unit quantities to minimize contamination of larger supplies.

All contaminated items are placed in sealed, sturdy biohazard bags and disposed of according to local, state and federal environmental regulations (ADA, 1996; CDC, 2003) (see Appendix A.2, Waste Management).

A.1.2 *Operative Procedures*

Gloves are worn during the performance of all intraoral radiographic procedures and when handling contaminated film packets, instruments, and other contaminated items, and during clean up procedures. Disposable gloves cannot be washed or decontaminated to be reused (ADA, 1996; Brand *et al.*, 1992; CDC, 2003; OSHA, 2001).

Gloves need not be worn while handling charts and paper work or mounting processed radiographs (Brand *et al.*, 1992).

Hands are washed before and after wearing gloves. Hands or skin are washed and mucous membranes flushed immediately or as soon as feasible after contact with blood or other potentially infectious materials, including saliva, in dental procedures (ADA, 1996; CDC, 2003; OSHA, 2001).

Either protective eyewear and masks or chin-length face shields are used during unusual radiographic procedures when splash or spatter is anticipated. Protective glasses need to have solid side-shields (ADA, 1996; CDC, 2003; OSHA, 2001). Since oral radiographic procedures generally do not result in splash or spatter, the use of these items may not be routinely required.

Protective clothing is required when exposure of skin or clothing to body fluids is anticipated. The type and characteristic of protective clothing will depend on the procedure and amount of exposure anticipated (ADA, 1996; OSHA, 2001).

A.1.3 *Darkroom Procedures*

Contaminated film packets are wiped dry and placed in a paper cup or other disposable container before proceeding to the darkroom (Brand *et al.*, 1992). Care should be taken not to contaminate the outer surface of the container. Contaminated gloves are removed and hands washed, or overgloves donned, prior to leaving the x-ray operatory to minimize the potential for contamination.

Gloves are required when handling contaminated film packets in the darkroom. Darkroom surfaces that may become contaminated are covered with an appropriate barrier or cleaned and disinfected following processing. Film packets are opened with gloved hands and films allowed to drop out of the packets without contamination. After disposing of the empty film packets, gloves are removed and films processed (ADA, 1996; Brand *et al.*, 1992).

An acceptable alternative involves enclosing the film packet in a barrier bag during exposure. After dropping the exposed film packet out of its barrier bag, gloves are removed before handling film and film packets for processing (ADA, 1996; Brand *et al.*, 1992).

Contamination of daylight-loading processors is difficult to avoid, and thus, their use is discouraged (Brand *et al.*, 1992). Processing of uncontaminated films, protected by barrier bags during exposure, will decrease the potential for contamination when using daylight loaders.

A.2 Waste Management

Presently, many states have passed laws or regulations governing the handling, storage and disposal of medical waste, as part of their overall hazardous waste program (EPA, 1986). Regulations concerning the handling and disposal of medical waste vary by location. Local and state regulations may be more restrictive than federal regulations, and should be consulted concerning the management of regulated and hazardous waste.

EPA recommends that facilities generating medical waste establish an infectious waste management plan (EPA, 1986). Local and state regulations should be consulted concerning the designation, handling and disposal of medical waste.

Items used during oral radiographic procedures that would release blood or other potentially infectious materials in a liquid or semiliquid state if compressed, or that are caked with dried blood or other potentially infectious materials and are capable of releasing such materials when handled, would be considered regulated waste (EPA, 1994; OSHA, 2001).

Regulated medical waste, including waste generated from dental radiographic procedures, is segregated from ordinary solid waste at the point of origin and placed in closable, leak-proof containers for handling, storage, transport or shipping. Containers are labeled with the biohazard label or color-coded red (EPA, 1986; OSHA, 2001). OSHA (2001) and EPA (1994) should be consulted concerning additional requirements for the management of contaminated sharps.

Regulated medical waste prepared for shipment are packaged in an appropriate container, which is rigid, leak-proof, impervious to moisture, tear-resistant, appropriately labeled, and sealed to prevent leakage (EPA, 1994). This waste is stored and disposed of according to local, state and federal regulations.

Waste may be identified as hazardous by consulting a list of hazardous wastes published in the Code of Federal Regulations (EPA, 1994), or in local and state regulations. Waste is considered hazardous if it exhibits one or more specified characteristics, including the presence of specified concentrations of certain toxic contaminants (EPA, 1994).

Spent film processing solutions containing silver in concentrations equal to or greater than five milligrams per liter are considered a hazardous waste when placed in containers and transported to a disposal site (EPA, 1994; Kodak, 1991).

Lead foil from dental film packets is a hazardous waste (EPA, 1994; Kodak, 1991). Lead foil is segregated from other solid waste following film processing, and disposed of according to local, state and federal regulations.

Film wash effluent is considered an industrial or commercial waste, and is disposed of through a municipal sewer system or septic tank system. When using a municipal sewer system, the effluent is considered to be effectively treated if the sewer system utilizes a secondary biological wastewater treatment plant. Local and state regulations should be consulted, as a discharge permit may be required. When a septic tank system is used, state or local regulations may dictate certain discharge permitting and monitoring requirements (Kodak, 1991).

The silver contained in film processing fixer solutions and wash water is often regulated by local and state discharge regulations. Regulations may require the recovery of silver from film processing solutions. Silver recovery through the processing of discarded radiographs and scrap film is encouraged (EPA, 1990; Kodak, 1991).

A.3 Hazardous Chemicals

A list of hazardous chemicals known to be present in the workplace should be compiled. OSHA (1994a) should be consulted concerning the determination of hazardous chemicals. Chemicals listed need to be identified in a manner in which they can be referenced on the appropriate material safety data sheet.

Incoming containers of hazardous chemicals are labeled, tagged or marked with the identity of the hazardous chemical, appropriate hazard warnings, and the manufacturer's name and address. Containers of hazardous chemicals in the workplace are labeled, tagged or marked with the identity of the hazardous chemical and appropriate hazard warnings. Exemptions may apply in certain situations as specified by OSHA (1994a).

A material safety data sheet is maintained for each hazardous chemical used in the workplace. Material safety data sheets need to be readily accessible to all employees. When hazards are determined to be present, or likely to be present in the workplace, the appropriate types of personal protective equipment are used to protect against the identified hazards. Personal protective equipment may include eye, face, head, foot and hand protection, depending on the identified hazard (OSHA, 1994b). Appropriate personal protective equipment is used in the darkroom to protect against exposure to film processing solutions and other harmful substances (AADR, 1983). Recommendations for quality assurance in dental radiography have been made by the Quality Assurance Committee of the American Academy of Oral and Maxillofacial Radiology (AADR, 1983).

Appendix B

Risk Assessment

Ionizing radiations and their biological effects have been one of the most intensively investigated areas of biomedical research. High-dose effects are well known and have been extensively published in both textbooks (*e.g.*, Hall, 1994; Mettler and Upton, 1995) and reviews by scientific bodies (ICRP, 1991; NAS/NRC, 1990; NCRP, 1993b; UNSCEAR, 2000). However, there remains uncertainty in the risk of harmful effects from very low doses, such as those encountered by patients and operators in dental radiography.

B.1 Stochastic Effects

These low-dose effects consist almost entirely of cancer and mutation. They are generally rare events, occurring only after a latent period of years to decades for cancer and generations for genetic effects. Thus, they present practical problems in the design of studies for their investigation. In the cohort of 86,572 Japanese atomic-bomb survivors there were 9,335 deaths from solid cancers between 1950 and 1997; only 440 were estimated to be excess over spontaneous incidence and thus attributable to radiation exposure (Preston *et al.*, 2003). Risks from low doses have been estimated by extrapolation from high-dose data (Brenner *et al.*, 2003; ICRP, 1991; NAS/NRC, 1990; NCRP, 1993b; Pierce and Preston, 2000; UNSCEAR, 1994, 2000). There has been considerable disagreement in the literature concerning the model used for such extrapolation. For radiation protection purposes, NCRP recommends use of the linear nonthreshold dose-response model for estimating the nominal risk of low doses (NCRP, 1993b).

B.1.1 *Cancer*

Excess cancer has been observed in many different organs and tissues in several irradiated human populations. The largest group, from which most quantitative data has come, is the Japanese atomic-bomb survivors. Data from this group and from patients treated with therapeutic radiation for a variety of both benign and malignant diseases, patients exposed to various types of diagnostic radiologic procedures, and groups exposed to occupational and environmental radiation have been extensively reviewed and analyzed (ICRP, 1991; NAS/NRC, 1990; NCRP, 1993b; UNSCEAR, 1994; 2000). Results have been frequently expressed as the probability of a health effect in an exposed population per unit dose. For example, a fatal cancer risk of 5 percent Sv^{-1} (see discussion on risk estimates in this Appendix) denotes a lifetime probability of one death from radiation-induced cancer in 20 individuals for a population where each individual received 1 Sv. Another way of expressing risk is to relate radiation effect to spontaneous risk. The lifetime probability of death from spontaneous cancer in the United States is about four in 20 individuals. Thus, for a population where each individual received a whole-body equivalent dose of 1 Sv, there would be an increase in the probability of death from cancer of one individual in 20 (*i.e.*, from four to five in 20). It should be noted, however, that doses to individuals in the U.S. population from dental x-ray procedures are on the order of microsieverts and millisieverts (*i.e.*, 10^{-6} and 10^{-3} Sv).

Available data for high doses (primarily the Japanese atomic-bomb survivor data) show an association between lifetime radiogenic cancer risk (incidence and death) and gender (Table B.1) (UNSCEAR, 2000). A similar association between lifetime risk of death and age at exposure was found for solid tumors but not for leukemia (Figure B.1) (UNSCEAR, 1994). UNSCEAR estimated the risk of exposure-induced death at 10.2 percent Sv^{-1} (UNSCEAR, 2000). A committee of the National Research Council estimated the overall risk of fatal cancer at 8 percent Sv^{-1} (NAS/NRC, 1990); ICRP estimated 9.5 percent Sv^{-1} (ICRP, 1991); and NCRP estimated 10 percent Sv^{-1} (NCRP, 1993b). All these estimates apply to an acute whole-body equivalent dose of 1 Sv delivered at a high-dose rate, and are averaged over both sexes and all ages. In general, effects from low-LET (linear-energy transfer) radiation are dependent on dose rate as well as dose. For radiation protection purposes, both the ICRP and NCRP have adopted a dose and dose-rate effectiveness factor of two for low-LET radiation. That is, risks per unit equivalent dose obtained for acute single doses should be divided by two to obtain an estimate of risks per unit dose for low-level or protracted exposures. Risk of fatal cancer from low-level (*e.g.*, diagnostic or environmental) radiation

TABLE B.1—*Site-specific risks for cancer incidence and mortality: U.S. population; relative risk model; acute whole-body equivalent dose of 1 Sv.*[a,b]

Site	Risk of Exposure-Induced			
	Incidence (percent)		Death (percent)	
	Males	Females	Males	Females
Esophagus	0.2	0.1	0.3	0.2
Stomach	0.2	0.1	0.1	0.2
Colon	1.1	1.9	0.9	1.9
Liver	0.1	0.1	0.2	0.2
Lung	2.9	7.5	3.1	3.2
Breast	0.0	13.6	0.0	5.2
Thyroid	0.4	0.5	—[c]	—[c]
Bladder	0.4	1.0	0.4	0.3
Other solid cancer	6.8	2.2	1.8	3.2
Leukemia	0.7	1.0	1.0	1.5
Total[d]	19.7	30.2	7.8	15.9

[a]Data in Table B.1 from UNSCEAR (2000). UNSCEAR presented estimates of lifetime risks of leukemia and solid cancers based on Japanese atomic-bomb survivor cancer mortality data (1950 to 1990) and cancer incidence data (1958 to 1987). Lifetime risks for mortality from all cancers were higher for females than males (Table B.1), and decreased with increasing age at exposure (*e.g.*, Figure B.1). Lifetime risks of leukemia were also higher for females than males (Table B.1), but showed little dependence on age at exposure (*e.g.*, Figure B.1) (data in Figure B.1 from UNSCEAR, 1994).

[b]UNSCEAR noted that discrepancies between incidence and death data for some organs occur because of differences in reference populations.

[c]Negligible.

[d]Total may differ from sum of individual values for each column because of rounding.

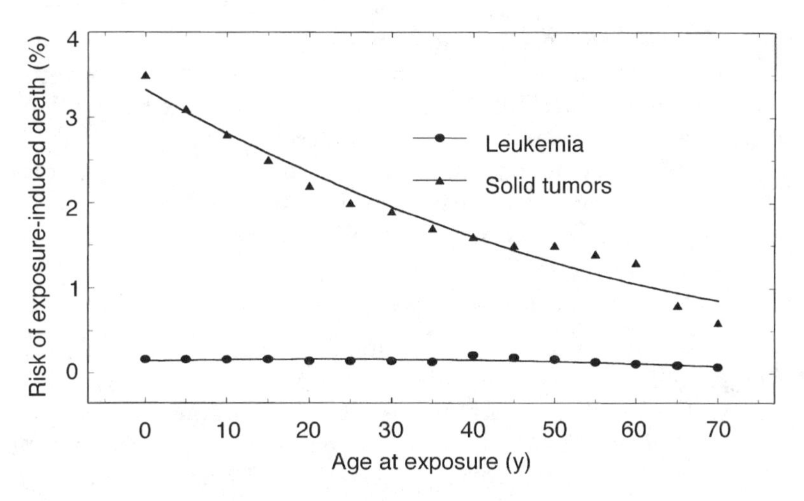

Fig. B.1. Risk of exposure-induced death from radiation-induced cancer by age at exposure at 200 mSv acute whole-body equivalent dose. Risk of solid tumors declines markedly with age at exposure while that of leukemia is essentially independent of age at exposure (UNSCEAR, 1994).

exposure is thus estimated at 4 to 6 percent Sv^{-1}. NCRP has previously pointed out the uncertainties in these risk estimates (NCRP, 1997). There is considerable uncertainty in applying this risk factor to doses less than 100 mSv (NCRP, 1993b). Doll and Wakeford (1997) reported an association between fetal doses of 10 mSv and increased risk of childhood cancer. Preston *et al.* (2003) showed increased cancer risk in Japanese atomic-bomb survivors at doses less than 50 mSv. However, Cohen (2002) cited evidence for decreased cancer of several types at low doses, suggesting a beneficial effect of such doses, but this finding is controversial (Puskin, 2003; Van Pelt, 2003). Although most epidemiological data are consistent with linear extrapolation, they are also compatible with other models of dose response relationships that would predict higher or lower risks at low doses.

The subject of carcinogenesis from prenatal exposure to radiation has been intensively studied since the first report of an association between prenatal diagnostic exposure and childhood cancer (Giles *et al.*, 1956). Numerous case-control epidemiologic studies have reported statistically significant associations between diagnostic exposure and childhood cancer, with relative risks at about 1.4 (Bithell, 1989). Nearly all cohort studies, on the other hand, have failed to find significant associations (Boice and Miller, 1999). No excess childhood cancers were detected in prenatally-exposed offspring of Japanese atomic-bomb survivors (Jablon and Kato, 1970). Excess adult-onset cancers were reported in this group (Delongchamp *et al.*, 1997); the risk was not significantly different from that for exposure of children. Recently, Doll and Wakeford (1997) have concluded that there is no threshold for radiation-induced cancer from exposure *in utero*, and that the risk is about 6 percent Gy^{-1} (absorbed dose in the embryo or fetus).

B.1.2 *Organs and Tissues Exposed by Dental X-Ray Procedures*

Organs and tissues in the head and neck that are included in the primary beam receive the principal exposure from dental x rays. The trunk and extremities receive only minor levels of scattered radiation. Absorbed doses to organs inferior to the diaphragm from dental radiology rarely exceed 1×10^{-3} mGy (Gibbs *et al.*, 1987; 1988b). Organs and tissues in the head and neck for which quantitative data for risk of radiation carcinogenesis exist (Table B.2) include active bone marrow, bone surfaces, skin, and thyroid. For each organ or tissue, these data apply to uniform exposure over that entire organ or tissue. Thus, the dose delivered to a part of a distributed tissue (such as active bone marrow) should be averaged over that entire tissue. Other organs or tissues included in the remainder in Table B.2, for which epidemiological data for radiation carcinogenesis exist, but for which quantitative risk remains uncertain include brain and meninges, epithelial lining of the paranasal sinuses, salivary glands, parathyroid glands, oral cavity, pharynx, and larynx (Boice *et al.*, 1996; Thompson *et al.*, 1994; UNSCEAR, 2000).

The spontaneous incidence of leukemia is quite small. Thus a small number of excess cases in an irradiated population constitutes a large relative risk (Shimizu *et al.*, 1990). The organ at risk for leukemia is active bone marrow. Epidemiologic studies have shown associations between diagnostic exposure (including dental) and leukemia (Graham *et al.*, 1966). About 16 percent of active bone marrow in healthy adults is found in the calvarium, mandible, and cervical vertebrae (Ellis, 1961). The dose delivered to the portion of the marrow in or near the primary beam is averaged over the entire marrow to generate the mean active bone marrow absorbed dose, which is used for computation of risk estimates. Active bone marrow absorbed dose from dental radiologic procedures ranges from 4×10^{-3} to 0.2 mGy (Gibbs *et al.*, 1987; 1988b).

Bone tumors, especially osteogenic sarcoma, are rare and occur following high-dose skeletal exposure to radium. There are no reliable data to estimate risks from external exposure. The risk is

TABLE B.2—*Nominal probability coefficients. Chronic exposure averaged over both sexes and all ages.*[a]

Tissue or Organ	Percent per Sievert (equivalent dose)			
	Fatal Cancer		Detriment[b]	
	Whole Population	Occupationally Exposed	Whole Population	Occupationally Exposed
Bladder	0.30	0.24	0.29	0.24
Active bone marrow	0.50	0.40	1.04	0.83
Bone surface	0.05	0.04	0.07	0.06
Breast	0.20	0.16	0.36	0.29
Colon	0.85	0.68	1.03	0.82
Esophagus	0.30	0.24	0.24	0.19
Liver	0.15	0.12	0.16	0.13
Lung	0.85	0.68	0.80	0.64
Ovary	0.10	0.08	0.15	0.12
Skin	0.02	0.02	0.04	0.03
Stomach	1.10	0.88	1.00	0.80
Thyroid	0.08	0.06	0.15	0.12
Remainder	0.50	0.40	0.59	0.47
Total	5.00	4.00	5.92	4.74
	Severe Hereditary Disorders			
Gonads	1.00	0.60	1.33	0.80
Total detriment (rounded)			7.3	5.6

[a]Data from ICRP (1991).
[b]See definition in Glossary and also see Appendix B.1.4.

greater in males than females and is inversely related to age at exposure (Mettler and Upton, 1995). No positive associations between diagnostic exposure and bone tumors have been reported. The dose to bone is averaged over the entire skeleton for risk estimation. Absorbed doses to bone surfaces from dental radiologic procedures range from 5×10^{-2} to 2 mGy (Gibbs *et al.*, 1987; 1988b).

Excess nonmelanoma skin cancers have been reported in a number of exposed populations, including multiple fluoroscopy of the chest, which delivered large accumulated doses in tuberculosis patients (Davis *et al.*, 1987). Excess basal cell cancer, but not squamous cell cancer or melanoma, has been reported in Japanese atomic-bomb survivors (Ron *et al.*, 1998). No tumors, however, have been seen following usual diagnostic doses. Since these tumors are now very curable, there may be a problem of underreporting. As with active bone marrow, absorbed dose to exposed skin is averaged over the entire skin. Dental x rays do not add significantly to the risk of skin cancer. Skin absorbed doses from dental radiology range from 7×10^{-3} to 0.4 mGy (Gibbs *et al.*, 1987; 1988b).

The juvenile thyroid is among the most radiosensitive organs to radiation-induced tumors, both benign and malignant. Ron *et al.* (1995) reported, from a pooled analysis of seven large-scale epidemiological studies of exposure to external radiation, a linear dose-response curve from exposure of children (age <15 y), with an excess relative risk per gray (thyroid absorbed dose) of 7.7. They found that risk decreased significantly with age at exposure, essentially disappearing after age 20. Early studies by Hempelmann *et al.* (1975) found that female infants were more sensitive than males, and certain racial or ethnic groups appeared more sensitive than the U.S. population at large. There is little evidence of risk from internal emitters. Studies of thyroid cancer from ^{131}I in fallout from early atmospheric tests of nuclear bombs in Nevada found significant associations only in those exposed within 1 y of birth and in the 1950 to 1959 birth cohort (Gilbert *et al.*, 1998). No overall statistically significant associations were detected. No thyroid cancers in excess of those attributable to pre-existing disease were found in patients given diagnostic exposure to ^{131}I (Hall *et al.*, 1996). In most studies, thyroid cancers induced by radiation have been low grade with long latent periods and rarely fatal (Mettler and Upton, 1995). Studies from Belarus and the Ukraine have found excess thyroid cancer in children exposed following the accident at Chernobyl (Jacob *et al.*, 1999). These tumors have been aggressive and began appearing in excess within 5 y after exposure (Kaul *et al.*, 1996). Some studies have reported excess thyroid cancer following therapeutic irradiation for tinea capitis in children, with mean thyroid absorbed doses of 90 mGy (Ron and Modan, 1984). Others, from similar exposures, found no excess thyroid cancer (Shore *et al.*, 1976). Absorbed doses to the thyroid from dental radiography range from 2×10^{-2} to 3 mGy (Gibbs *et al.*, 1987; 1988b).

Excess brain cancer has been identified in two series of patients treated for tinea capitis (Ron and Modan, 1984; Shore *et al.*, 1976) and in numerous studies of high-dose radiotherapy. No statistically significant excess of brain cancer has been detected in the Japanese atomic-bomb survivors or in several studies of occupationally-exposed workers. However, an analysis of all nervous system tumors (including benign tumors) has shown a statistically significant dose response in Japanese atomic-bomb survivors (Preston *et al.*, 2002). An association of both brain and meningeal tumors with dental x ray has been identified, but statistical significance is marginal (Preston-Martin *et al.*, 1989). Another study failed to confirm the association with gliomas (Burch *et al.*, 1987). Karlsson *et al.* (1998) reported a linear dose-response curve for intracranial tumors following exposure of infants to a mean intracranial absorbed dose of 70 mGy. They found an excess relative risk per gray of 4.5 for first exposure before age five months, 1.5 at ages five to seven months, and 0.4 thereafter. Brain absorbed doses from dental radiology are 5×10^{-3} to 0.16 mGy (Gibbs *et al.*, 1987; 1988b).

Radiation association with cancer of the epithelial lining of the paranasal sinuses has been identified only from internally-deposited ^{226}Ra (Rowland and Lucas, 1984), at a cumulative lifetime risk level of 6.4 excess carcinomas per million exposed per millisievert (equivalent dose). Radium is metabolized in the same manner as calcium, a bone seeker. Radium-226 deposited in the facial skeleton decays to ^{222}Rn, a radioactive gas that accumulates in the sinus cavities and exposes the epithelium. The sinus epithelium receives absorbed doses of 5×10^{-2} to 4.6 mGy from dental radiology (Gibbs *et al.*, 1987; 1988b).

Excess incidence of both benign and malignant tumors of the salivary glands has been reported in the Japanese atomic-bomb survivors (Boice *et al.*, 1996; Thompson *et al.*, 1994), and in several studies of children treated with therapeutic radiation for benign disease (Modan *et al.*, 1977). Excess relative risk per sievert (equivalent dose in the salivary glands) has ranged from 0.1 to 0.7 (Boice *et al.*, 1996). An association with dental x rays has been reported (Preston-Martin *et al.*, 1988). Absorbed doses to salivary glands from dental radiologic procedures range from 0.1 to 5.5 mGy (Gibbs *et al.*, 1987; 1988b).

Radiation has been implicated in the etiology of parathyroid tumors in several studies of patients following therapeutic irradiation for benign disease (Mettler and Upton, 1995). Hyperparathyroidism has been detected in several of these studies and in the Japanese atomic-bomb survivors (Takeichi *et al.*, 1991). The interrelationship of these tumors with other endocrine abnormalities has not been clearly defined in several of these studies. Parathyroid absorbed doses from dental radiology are similar to those to the thyroid, 2×10^{-2} to 3 mGy.

Slight excesses, not statistically significant, in tumors of the oral cavity, pharynx, and larynx have been found in atomic-bomb survivors (Ron *et al.*, 1994). No excess has been detected in numerous studies of occupationally-exposed workers and patients exposed to diagnostic radiation, nuclear medicine, or treated with therapeutic radiation for various diseases (Mettler and Upton, 1995). Extreme care must be taken in interpreting the positive results because of the well-known cofactors, alcohol and tobacco abuse. It is not clear that there is any statistically significant association, and no risk factors are available. Absorbed doses to these tissues from dental radiology range up to 5 mGy (Gibbs *et al.*, 1987; 1988b).

B.1.3 *Genetic Effects*

Analysis of data from a population of more than 30,000 offspring of Japanese atomic-bomb survivors for several indicators of hereditary disease (untoward pregnancy outcome, childhood death, childhood cancer, chromosomal abnormalities, abnormal protein metabolism, sex ratio, and physical development of the child) has failed to detect a statistically significant effect (UNSCEAR, 1993).

Excess incidence of leukemia in children of workers at one nuclear plant in the United Kingdom has been reported (Gardner *et al.*, 1990). These results suggested that effective doses as low as 10 mSv, delivered at low dose rates to fathers, may cause a large increase in leukemia in their children. However, these findings, on careful analysis, result from four cases; they are also inconsistent with all other human experience. The report triggered additional studies in offspring of several irradiated populations, all with basically negative results (UNSCEAR, 1993).

Using multisite DNA fingerprinting, Weinberg *et al.* (2001) reported a sevenfold increase in new DNA bands in offspring of Chernobyl cleanup workers, compared to siblings born before the Chernobyl accident and to offspring of unexposed families.

However, Livshits *et al.* (2001) found no significant increase in mutation rates in minisatellite alleles in the same population. They did see an increase, not statistically significant, in offspring conceived within two months of exposure of the father in the cleanup operations, as compared to those born later of the same parents.

The nature and magnitude of genetic effects of radiation in human populations remains unclear. UNSCEAR (2001) has suggested a doubling dose of 0.82 ± 0.29 Gy (absorbed dose in the parental gonads), which UNSCEAR rounds to 1 Gy for risk estimation.

Current estimates show that genetic risk from dental radiation is numerically smaller than cancer risk. Gonadal absorbed doses from common dental exposures are too small to measure accurately and are frequently neglected in dental dosimetry studies. Computer simulations of radiation transport from dental x-ray sources have estimated gonadal absorbed doses of less than 1×10^{-4} mGy per full-mouth intraoral or panoramic examination (Gibbs *et al.*, 1988a; 1988b). The gonadal equivalent dose to the average American from naturally-occurring environmental sources is about 0.9 mSv y^{-1} (NCRP, 1987a). Thus the gonadal absorbed dose from a typical dental x-ray procedure is equivalent to about 1 h of natural background radiation.[1] The genetically significant dose from all diagnostic radiation exposure in the healing arts was estimated at 0.3 mGy y^{-1} for the United States in 1980. The contribution to genetically significant dose from dental radiation is less than 1×10^{-3} mGy y^{-1} and is excluded from the computation (NCRP, 1989c).

B.1.4 *Effective Dose*

In 1977, ICRP introduced the term detriment, which is a weighted probability of stochastic effect (ICRP, 1977), and further expanded the concept in 1990 (ICRP, 1991). Detriment is a complex concept that includes fatal and nonfatal cancer, genetic effects, and loss of life span from cancer and hereditary disease; it also is weighted for severity and time of expression of the harmful effect. ICRP estimated a detriment of 7.3 percent Sv^{-1} for uniform whole-body equivalent dose at a low dose rate to the whole population,

[1]Since the value of the radiation weighting factor for dental x rays is assigned the value of one, gonadal absorbed dose and gonadal equivalent dose are numerically equal.

and 5.6 percent Sv^{-1} for the occupationally-exposed population. The detriment is averaged over both sexes and all ages in the respective populations (Table B.2). NCRP concurred with these estimates (NCRP, 1993b).

A major problem in the evaluation of risk from radiation exposure in the healing arts is the nonuniform dose distribution in both patients and occupationally-exposed personnel. One method of estimating this risk is to determine the equivalent dose to each susceptible organ, multiply that dose by its specific organ nominal probability coefficient (Table B.2), and sum the results for total risk. Another approach is a method called effective dose equivalent by Jacobi (1975), which was adopted by the ICRP (1977). A similar somatic dose index was proposed by Laws and Rosenstein (1978). The method estimated the uniform whole-body equivalent dose that would carry the same probability of stochastic effect as the nonuniform equivalent doses actually received by the relevant organs and tissues. It is accomplished by modifying the equivalent dose to each susceptible organ by a tissue weighting factor determined from the relative contribution of detriment from that organ to total detriment. Although initially intended for use only in radiation protection from occupational exposure, the method has been used to compare relative radiation doses for a variety of situations, including diagnostic exposure in patients. In 1990, ICRP revised and updated the method, and renamed it effective dose (E) (ICRP, 1991), computed as:

$$E = \Sigma w_T H_T, \qquad \text{(B.1)}$$

where H_T is the equivalent dose in tissue or organ T and w_T is the tissue weighting factor for that tissue (Table B.3). The effective dose from one type of exposure can be compared to that from some other type of exposure, such as the effective dose from natural sources, about 3 mSv y^{-1} in the United States (NCRP, 1987a).

There remains a high level of uncertainty in the numeric values of detriment and tissue weighting factors. For radiogenic cancer, the uncertainty arises from at least four factors (NCRP, 1993b): (1) the choice of any given risk projection model among several that fit available data almost equally well, (2) the duration of excess risk following a given exposure, (3) application of risk factors derived from high doses at high dose rates to low doses protracted over time, and (4) the extrapolation of risk factors from one population to another having differing incidences of specific tumors or cancer in general. For genetic effects, the absence of human data showing

TABLE B.3—*Tissue weighting factors.*[a]

Tissue or Organ	Tissue Weighting Factor
Gonads	0.20
Bone marrow (red)	0.12
Colon	0.12
Lung	0.12
Stomach	0.12
Bladder	0.05
Breast	0.05
Esophagus	0.05
Liver	0.05
Thyroid	0.05
Skin	0.01
Bone surface	0.01
Remainder[b]	0.05

[a]Developed from a reference population of equal numbers of both sexes and a wide age range; applicable to both workers and the population at large (data from ICRP, 1991).

[b]Composed of adrenals, brain, upper large intestine, small intestine, kidney, muscle, pancreas, spleen, thymus, and uterus.

a statistically significant increase in hereditary disease in offspring of exposed populations places total dependence on the results from animal studies.

As used in radiation protection, detriment and effective dose apply to an average individual in a population (*i.e.*, detriment and effective dose have been formulated for a population of both sexes and all ages) and cannot be used to estimate radiation risk to a specific individual. Risk of radiogenic cancer is dependent on age and sex of the exposed person or persons. Risk of genetic effects disappears in females at menopause and declines with age in males, paralleling the decrease in probability of fathering additional offspring. These known dependencies of tissue weighting factors on age and sex make comparisons of effective doses subject to error when age and sex distributions of the populations differ.

It is clear that estimates of risk for stochastic effects from ionizing radiation have changed over time, as new information became available. It is likely that concepts of risk and estimates of its magnitude will continue to evolve as more extensive and more accurate data become available.

B.2 Deterministic Effects

When sufficient numbers of functional parenchymal cells in a given organ or tissue are killed, then the function of that organ or tissue may be impaired or destroyed. If that function is vital, then the injury may be life threatening to the organism. These effects, called deterministic effects, occur in those individuals for whom the dose is sufficient, *i.e.*, greater than some threshold. Acute deterministic effects (*i.e.*, radiation syndrome) have been seen in several populations days to weeks after exposure (Hall, 1994; Rubin and Casarett, 1968; UNSCEAR, 1993). Recently, other deterministic effects (diseases of circulatory, digestive and respiratory systems) have been detected in Japanese atomic-bomb survivors after long latent periods (Preston *et al.*, 2003; Shimizu *et al.*, 1999). At subthreshold doses cells may be killed but at a clinically insignificant level. These effects follow large radiation doses (absorbed doses of the order of grays and higher) and will not be encountered in the use of dental diagnostic radiation.

B.2.1 *Effects in the Embryo and Fetus*

Human pregnancy is typically divided into three periods: (1) preimplantation-implantation, approximately the first two weeks after conception, during which the major activity is rapid cell division; (2) major organogenesis, weeks three through seven, when most differentiation occurs; and (3) the fetal period, from the eighth week through term, characterized by rapid growth of the fetus (Brent, 1999). Consensus data from rodent experiments and human experience indicate that the only effect from radiation exposure during the preimplantation period is prenatal death of the embryo; the threshold absorbed dose is about 0.1 Gy on day zero, increasing thereafter. Congenital anomalies and neonatal death may follow exposure during major organogenesis. Most experts cite an estimated threshold absorbed dose of 0.2 Gy (Brent, 1999); a few animal experiments have found effects at absorbed doses of 5×10^{-2} Gy. NCRP has concluded that statistically significant increases in incidence of congenital anomalies require absorbed doses in excess of 0.15 Gy (NCRP, 1977). Radiation-induced anomalies mimic those that occur spontaneously; they occur in organs or tissues that were at a critical period in development or differentiation at the time of exposure.

Growth retardation and mental retardation may occur from exposure postimplantation. The period of maximum sensitivity for severe mental retardation is the eighth through fifteenth week postovulation. In offspring of Japanese atomic-bomb survivors exposed to 1 Gy (absorbed dose in the embryo or fetus) during this period the frequency of severe mental retardation was 40 percent (background frequency 0.8 percent), with IQ reduced by 25 points, and average school performance reduced from the 50th to the lower 10th percentile. Sensitivity appeared lower during the 16 to 25 week period, and was essentially absent before eight weeks and after 25 weeks. Sensitivity to radiation-induced small head size also varied with gestational age at exposure; the maximum was at 8 to 15 weeks, followed by zero to seven weeks, with 16 weeks to term showing minimum sensitivity. Small head size was more than twice as frequent as severe mental retardation in this population. About half of the severely retarded individuals also had small head size. It should be emphasized that the data for severe metal retardation and small head size are not yet sufficient to establish risk estimates for absorbed doses in the embryo or fetus below about 0.5 Gy (UNSCEAR, 1993).

B.2.2 *Exposure to the Embryo and Fetus in Dental X-Ray Procedures*

There is always concern when exposure of a female who is pregnant, but not aware of it, occurs. Such exposure happens occasionally during very early, unrecognized pregnancy. The absorbed dose to the embryo or fetus from dental x ray is small, similar to gonadal absorbed dose and well below the threshold for deterministic effects. If x-ray exposure is required for adequate diagnosis and treatment for a pregnant person, then the radiologic procedure should be conducted so as to minimize the radiation dose to the pelvic region. If dental care is to be delayed until after delivery, then exposure should also be delayed. Common dental projections rarely, if ever, deliver a measurable absorbed dose to the embryo or fetus.

Appendix C

Evaluation of Radiation Safety Program Performance and Equipment Performance

This Appendix deals with setting up and evaluating programs for protection of workers and members of the public from sources of radiation used in dentistry. Protection of the patient is considered explicitly in Section 3. However, it should always be kept in mind that any measure that reduces patient dose also reduces dose to workers and the public. For example, use of more sensitive image receptors reduces occupational exposure by reducing workload [milliampere-minutes per week (mA min week^{-1})]. Similarly, the implementation of a quality-assurance program may reduce repeat procedures, which also reduces workload and occupational exposure.

Although this Appendix deals with the major aspects of radiation protection programs, other references should also be consulted. Individuals seeking greater detail on the general principles of radiation protection should review NCRP Report No. 57 "*Instrumentation and Monitoring Methods for Radiation Protection*" (NCRP, 1978), Report No. 107 "*Implementation of the Principle of as Low as Reasonably Achievable (ALARA) for Medical and Dental Personnel*" (NCRP, 1990), Report No. 127 "*Operational Radiation Safety Program*" (NCRP, 1998), and Report No. 134 "*Operational Radiation Safety Training*" (NCRP, 2000).

C.1 Methods of Radiation Protection in Dentistry

A radiation protection program is an ongoing system of procedures, evaluation and monitoring applied to all aspects of design, construction, installation and use of radiation sources such that goals and criteria of radiation protection are met. Thus, while shielding design is an important aspect of radiation protection, a radiation protection program is more than just the provision of appropriate shielding. A dental radiation protection program considers all aspects of the use of x rays in a dental environment. This includes evaluation of categories of individuals who may be exposed to radiation and factors that affect individual exposure, as well as evaluation of how equipment design and performance, facility design and shielding, and operating procedures affect radiation exposure. In the presence of adequately designed shielding, the level of occupational exposure is primarily dependent upon adequate training of staff and careful observance of radiation protection procedures.

C.1.1 *Categories of Individuals to be Protected*

The radiation protection program needs to consider the categories of individuals to be protected. Protective barriers are designed for each specific category of protected individuals. Other possible protective measures, such as radiation protection education and training, also vary by category. For instance, an ongoing program of training (NCRP, 2000) in specific radiation protection procedures is essential for dental workers, but difficult (if not impossible) for members of the public.

C.1.1.1 *Occupationally-Exposed Individuals.* NCRP (1998) defines occupational exposure as "exposures to individuals that are incurred in the workplace as the result of situations that can be reasonably regarded as being the responsibility of management (exposures associated with medical diagnosis or treatment are excluded)." A worker need not be measurably exposed to radiation, nor individually monitored for level of radiation exposure to be considered occupationally exposed. As discussed in Appendix C.3, individual monitoring is based on the likelihood of receiving an effective dose greater than 1 mSv y^{-1}. EPA examined patterns of occupational exposure among U.S. dental workers (Kumazawa *et al.*, 1984), and found that the average annual effective dose equivalent (H_E)[2] was 0.2 mSv. Only 32 percent of U.S. dental workers received a measurable exposure during the period examined

[2]At the time, these data were reported in the quantity effective dose equivalent (H_E).

(calendar year 1980). Of those dental workers receiving some measurable exposure, the average annual value of H_E was 0.7 mSv. Thus, the majority of dental workers would not be expected to require individual monitoring. Nevertheless, dental workers are occupationally exposed to radiation. Any dental staff member who performs or assists in dental radiography should be considered to be occupationally exposed.

Pregnant employees are a special category of occupationally-exposed individuals. As discussed in Section 2, equivalent dose limits apply to the embryo and fetus, and limits are placed also on the equivalent dose per month. The shielding design goal for controlled areas (0.1 mGy week^{-1} air kerma) recommended in this Report for dental facilities would allow pregnant workers continued access to their work areas (NCRP, in press). In many states, additional radiation monitoring is required for pregnant employees. Special consideration also needs to be given to employees and students under 18 y of age (see Table 1.1 footnote).

C.1.1.2 *Nonoccupationally-Exposed Individuals.* Individuals not occupationally exposed, and not receiving radiation as a patient, are categorized as members of the public. In the context of dental practice, members of the public include workers in adjacent (nondental) office space, employees in the dental office not likely to be exposed to radiation as part of their normal duties (*e.g.*, a receptionist), and patients and their families in waiting areas. With "open space" architectural design, several patients may be separated by thin partitions or other radiolucent barriers. In such cases, a patient subject to primary and secondary radiation from another patient's imaging procedure is considered as a member of the public.

C.1.1.3 *Patients.* For purposes of radiation protection and tabulation of occupational and nonoccupational doses, the radiation dose received as a patient in the course of a medical or dental procedure is not included. This is because the individual patient receives direct benefit from the utilization of radiation. In the case of dental radiography, this benefit arises from the diagnostic information gained from the imaging procedure. Although there are no patient dose limits, the amount of patient radiation exposure should always be optimized to the minimum amount required to achieve the medical objective of the procedure. Typical patient doses and methods of patient dose reduction were discussed in Section 3.

For a given level of shielding, reduction of patient dose is always an effective method of reducing occupational and nonoccupational dose. Conversely, for a given level of occupational dose, reduction of patient dose reduces barrier thickness requirements.

C.1.2 *Protection by Equipment Design*

Equipment design effects radiation protection directly, by controlling primary and secondary radiation, and indirectly, by controlling patient dose. Some equipment design features, such as the thickness of lead in the x-ray tube housing, are determined at the time of manufacture and cannot be modified by the individual user. Other equipment features, such as collimator type and image receptor holder type, are user selectable. Specific design recommendations and performance standards for dental x-ray machines were discussed in Section 4.

Calculation of barrier thickness requires specific knowledge of equipment specifications. As part of the equipment documentation, the manufacturer is required to supply:

- x-ray generator waveform
- kVp range
- milliampere range
- timer range
- inherent and added filtration
- typical half-value layer at one or more values of kVp
- kVp and milliampere values used to determine x-ray tube head leakage
- measured average x-ray tube head leakage in mGy h^{-1} (or R h^{-1}) at a specified distance from the x-ray tube head
- dimensions and lead equivalence of all cones and collimators supplied with the equipment
- the presence and lead equivalence of shielding incorporated into image receptor holders that may act as a primary barrier.

Design of radiation protection policies and procedures also requires knowledge of equipment design, operation and safety features. The manufacturer supplies an operator's manual that describes the function of all controls, interlocks and safety features, and provides normal operating procedures. It is the responsibility of the user to ensure that adequate and current documentation of equipment specifications and operating procedures is maintained for all radiation producing equipment.

C.1.3 *Protection by Facility Design*

Radiation protection is provided by appropriate design and shielding of facilities used to perform dental radiography. Protection is provided not only by adequate radiation barrier thickness, but also by controlling access to and flow through areas used for imaging procedures. (Specific methods of barrier thickness calculation are discussed in Appendix F.) Layout of the overall facility also can affect radiation exposure by controlling occupancy of adjacent areas. A typical small office for general dentistry may consist of several operatory suites, a laboratory, a dark room, one or two private offices, a business office, and a patient waiting area. Intraoral radiography may be available in all operatory suites, but a small office would typically not contain more than one panoramic unit. A large dental practice or academic facility may have many operatory suites, some of which are dedicated only to dental imaging procedures. Radiation protection needs to be considered during the architectural design phase of dental facilities. Although it is often possible to shield a dental facility using conventional construction materials, and it may turn out that normal office construction provides adequate shielding, a radiation shielding design study should be performed by a qualified expert for all new construction and for significant x-ray equipment changes in existing facilities.

The architect and the qualified expert should work together to integrate the use of materials, room adjacencies, room occupancies, and distances to provide appropriate shielding while allowing efficient utilization of equipment and personnel and providing for the comfort and privacy of the patient. Various authors (Malkin, 2002; NCRP, in press) have discussed architectural considerations in the design of dental and medical x-ray facilities. Centralized design often is used to minimize travel distances, improve access, and allow fewer staff to cover more operatories. Corridors and other low occupancy spaces, such as rest rooms or utility rooms, may be used to separate radiation areas from occupied spaces such as offices and lounges. In the past, dental radiography rooms have been designed without a specific control booth. However, a shielded location allowing continuous visual observation of the patient is required for the dental x-ray machine operator.

So-called "open space" design may result in several operatory areas being separated by modular cabinets or thin mobile partitions. This design presents radiation protection problems. For this reason, it is discouraged. Careful attention to shielding design is required. Even in the absence of open space design, operatory suites may have door-less entries and windows on exterior walls.

For designs of this type, special consideration should be given to individuals occupying the adjacent operatory and individuals passing by unshielded openings. For instance, patients in open space operatories should be located such that they are not irradiated by the primary beam from an adjacent patient.

C.1.4 *Protection by Operating Procedure Design*

Equipment and facility radiation protection design criteria alone are insufficient to implement a radiation protection program. Radiation protection policies and procedures need to be developed for each dental facility. The recommendations of this Report, other professional guidelines, statutory requirements (*i.e.*, state radiation protection laws), and manufacturer's operation procedures are integrated into a set of local policies and procedures. The procedures need to be clearly written in language readily understood by the average employee, kept in an accessible format and location, and reviewed by all staff annually.

C.2 Radiation Protection Surveys, Documentation and Reporting

In this Report, radiation protection survey means an evaluation by a qualified expert of potential radiation exposure from the use of dental x-ray equipment under the specific conditions of a particular installation. Methods of radiation protection surveys for a variety of circumstances and institutions have been discussed in NCRP Report No. 57 (NCRP, 1978). In general, a complete radiation protection survey of a dental facility includes the following phases:

1. *Investigation*. Information is collected and examined regarding the facility design, including original shielding design study (if any), current architectural drawings showing layout and construction of barriers, the type, location and workload of all x-ray equipment, manufacturers documentation concerning radiation protection features and specifications of x-ray equipment, and applicable written radiation protection policies and procedures.
2. *Inspection*. The qualified expert personally verifies the presence of the x-ray equipment and investigates its condition and use, the operability and integrity of physical

safeguards, and the adherence of personnel to established procedures.

3. *Measurement*. Radiation measurements are obtained to evaluate the performance of x-ray equipment to assess typical radiation hazards during routine operation of equipment and to assess adequacy of radiation barriers.
4. *Evaluation*. The results of the inspection and measurements are converted into a form that can be directly compared with applicable shielding design goals or effective dose limits. The results of this comparison, together with the information obtained during the inspection, form the basis for an evaluation of the radiation protection status of the installation, and for recommendations regarding remedial action and resurvey after corrective action has been taken.

C.2.1 *Facility Surveys*

The purpose of a facility survey is to assess radiation protection features provided in the design and construction of the rooms containing dental x-ray equipment. The starting point for facility assessment is a review of the original architectural design and drawings, including the original report of shielding design. If no such documents and drawings exist, the qualified expert provides approximate drawings of the imaging procedure rooms and attempts to determine the material, construction and thickness of existing barriers. For a new facility, no design yet exists. In this case, a facility design study (*i.e.*, shielding design, layout and flow for optimal radiation protection) is performed by a qualified expert in conjunction with the architect. The facility survey indicates the location of equipment, location of physical safeguards such as control booths or portable shields, the degree of occupancy of all areas adjacent to radiation areas, and classification of persons exposed there as occupationally or nonoccupationally exposed.

The purpose of a facility radiation survey is to measure radiation levels at various locations and to compare these measurements with expected levels. The original shielding design report should indicate maximum instantaneous air-kerma rate (mGy h^{-1}) and average air-kerma rate (milligray per week) for specific locations within the facility. The qualified expert selects radiation detection instrumentation appropriate for the dental x-ray environment. Although area surveys may be performed with a sensitive electronically read instrument, such as a large volume high-pressure gas ionization survey meter, some instruments are relatively insensitive. Care should be taken to ensure that the instrument accurately detects expected radiation levels, particularly when assessing barrier transmission. If circumstances permit, film, thermoluminescent, or similar dosimeters (from a commercial service, for instance) may offer the best means of performing an area survey (Appendix C.3.1).

C.2.2 *Equipment Surveys*

The purpose of the equipment survey is to assess operational and protective features of dental radiographic equipment that can affect patient and operator exposure. The qualified expert first reviews available equipment documentation and performs the indicated measurements. During review of equipment documentation, the qualified expert ascertains and records the make and model of the equipment (both generator and x-ray tube), visible serial numbers of major components, date of manufacture, generator waveform, and kVp, milliampere, and timer ranges. The manufacturer's information on x-ray tube housing leakage radiation is reviewed. For equipment manufactured since 1978 it is not generally necessary to perform a leakage radiation survey unless there is reason to suspect that original housing shielding may have been compromised.

C.2.2.1 *Intraoral Equipment.* The qualified expert determines that the minimum distance from the target to the end of the cone is at least 20 cm and that the field size at the end of the cone is restricted to the limits discussed in Section 4. The type of collimation (circular versus rectangular, use of special collimation, etc.) is noted. Indicated and measured kVp and exposure time are required to agree within five percent or meet the manufacturer's specifications, whichever is more restrictive. Radiation output of the machine is measured using a calibrated ionization chamber or other appropriate device suitable for use with small beams of radiation. The entire sensitive volume of the chamber needs to fit within the radiation field. Radiation output per unit tube current (in units of mGy mAs^{-1} or mR mAs^{-1}) is measured at a specified location, such as the end of the cone, for the clinically useful range of kVp. These data, combined with typical technique factors, are used to calculate typical patient entrance air kerma or entrance skin exposure from various intraoral projections. The half-value layer is determined and compared to standards given by the FDA and appropriate state regulations.

C.2.2.2 *Panoramic Equipment*. The qualified expert confirms the presence of collimating slits and primary beam shielding as part of the image-receptor holder. The collimating slits are aligned within the limits discussed in Section 4. Although not necessary for radiation protection purposes, the qualified expert is advised to evaluate the motion of the unit to ensure that it is smooth and unimpeded. For machines used for both panoramic and cephalometric radiography, the qualified expert should also determine that the x-ray tube head locks in appropriate positions for each type of radiography, and that its position remains stable.

C.2.3 *Administrative Controls*

The purpose of an operational survey is to evaluate policies, procedures and training to assess whether radiation protection practices are observed during routine use of dental x-ray sources. The qualified expert reviews the policy and procedure manual, identifies the date of its last revision, assesses whether or not policies reflect current equipment and staffing, and compares local policies and procedures with statutory and professional standards. The qualified expert determines the adequacy of instruction of new employees in radiation protection and equipment operation, as well as that for existing employees obtaining continuing education. Facility and individual monitoring records are reviewed and exposure patterns assessed. Efforts to optimize radiation protection through the ALARA principle are reviewed. The presence of up-to-date technique charts and patient dose charts is confirmed.

C.3 Radiation Monitoring in Dentistry

C.3.1 *Facility Monitoring*

Facility monitoring is the routine measurement of radiation exposure levels at various fixed locations within a radiation area. Facility monitoring can serve several purposes. It can be used on a one-time basis to demonstrate the adequacy of shielding design and construction. It can be used on an ongoing basis to monitor the radiation environment to assess change or indicate need for additional protective measures. Finally, in certain circumstances, it can be used to estimate levels of individual exposure either in conjunction with or in lieu of a program of individual monitoring.

Facility monitoring can be carried out using the same types of radiation dosimeters [*i.e.*, film, thermoluminescent or optically-stimulated luminescent (OSL) dosimetry] used for individual monitoring. However, film dosimetry cannot be used over extended periods for area monitoring. When ordering dosimeters it is advisable to inform the dosimetry service of their intended use and to have facility dosimeters identified by name (*e.g.*, Monitor 1, Monitor 2, etc.) to avoid confusion with individual (personal) dosimeters. For evaluation of shielding integrity, dosimeters are placed on both sides of a barrier. For ongoing area monitoring, it is sufficient to locate a dosimeter inside each procedure room at the location of expected maximum exposure (usually the wall lateral to patient orientation) and to locate additional dosimeters in the areas where the operator stands while initiating an exposure.

Area dosimeters are left in place for a sufficient period to accumulate a measurable exposure. Reid and MacDonald (1984) monitored integrated exposure patterns during routine intraoral radiography over a five and a half month period in which 2,100 films were used. Readings on the lateral walls ranged from 0.18 to 1.05 mGy air kerma (20 to 120 mR exposure). MacDonald *et al.* (1983) suggested that a typical "busy" intraoral unit might use 180 films per week. Since the minimum detectable level for commercial thermoluminescent dosimeters is approximately 100 μSv (10 mrem) [10 μSv (1 mrem) for OSL dosimeters], periods in excess of one month often are required to obtain measurable readings. Depending on workload and location of dosimeters, a three or six month interval is suggested for intraoral dental facility monitoring. For panoramic units even longer intervals may be required. The data of Reid *et al.* (1993) indicate that 1 m from a panoramic unit, the average air kerma is approximately 0.45 μGy per exposure. Thus, about 222 exposures are required to exceed the threshold of detection for thermoluminescent dosimeters (about 22 exposures for OSL dosimeters).

C.3.2 *Personal Monitoring*

Measurements of the radiation exposure received by occupationally-exposed individuals serve two different purposes. They provide information that may lead to the identification of undesirable practices and of unsuspected sources of high exposure, thus permitting the prompt application of controls to limit such exposure (NCRP, 1990). They also provide some information regarding the exposure of the individual, permitting a demonstration of compliance with individual dose limits and documentation of annual and lifetime dose.

NCRP recommends that all occupationally-exposed persons who may receive an occupational effective dose of more than 1 mSv y^{-1} need to be individually monitored. State law may require individual monitoring of those who may receive more than 1/10 of the applicable dose limit. It may be more important, and is certainly prudent practice, to provide personal dosimeters for pregnant employees who may be occupationally exposed, because of the limit for equivalent dose to the embryo and fetus of 0.5 mSv in a month, once pregnancy is known. Individual monitoring is not required where the nature of the work performed or the nature of the radiation sources is such that exposures to personnel are below limits recommended for the general public and where there is a very small potential for accidental exposure above these limits. The decision of whether or not to individually monitor employees is based on applicable state law, as well as expected exposure patterns predicted on the basis of workload and available protective measures. If individual monitoring is not performed, facility monitoring needs to be performed.

Dose limits for stochastic effects are expressed in effective dose (Appendix G). Hence, for sophisticated calculations, explicit consideration is given to effects on organ dose of nonuniform exposure patterns due to small collimated radiation fields, and effects of tissue attenuation. Personal and facility dosimeters do not directly measure effective dose, although for uniform whole-body exposure, conversion factors may be derived to convert dosimeter readings to effective dose equivalents or effective doses (ICRP, 1988; 1996b). de Haan and van Aken (1990) have investigated effective dose equivalent to the operator in intraoral radiography.[3] Taking into account operator position and tissue attenuation, but omitting some collimation and image receptor attenuation effects, these authors calculated an effective dose equivalent to an operator standing 1 m from the patient to vary between 7.4×10^{-3} and 0.10 mSv per radiograph for D-speed film and between 4×10^{-3} and 6×10^{-2} mSv per radiograph for E-speed film (at 60 kVp in both cases). From their data, one can infer an approximate conversion factor from ambient exposure level at 1 m to effective dose equivalent of approximately 5×10^{-3} mSv mR^{-1}. Thus, at 60 kVp, a personal dosimeter worn at the location on the body of maximum exposure, would overestimate effective dose equivalent from intraoral radiography by about 70 percent. In general, conversion

[3]The quantity reported in de Haan and van Aken (1990) was effective dose equivalent. The quantity effective dose was not yet in use.

from a personal dosimeter reading to effective dose equivalent (or effective dose) is highly dependent on x-ray energy, collimation, and degree of nonuniformity of radiation exposure.

For nonuniform exposure patterns such as those encountered from tightly collimated beams of radiation, the position at which the personal dosimeter is located on the individual can complicate conversion of the dosimeter reading to effective dose. The personal dosimeter should be worn at the maximally exposed location on the body. Since the x-ray tube head is most often positioned at the head of a sitting patient, a personal dosimeter worn at the belt to chest level of a standing worker will receive the greatest exposure.

Past studies of occupational exposure patterns of dental workers have indicated that most dental workers would receive less than minimum detectable or very low (less than 1 mSv y^{-1}) annual occupational dose (Kumazawa *et al.*, 1984). For facilities that have low workloads, greater accuracy and reduced cost can be achieved by replacing personal dosimeters at greater than one-month intervals. However, excessive intervals do not allow timely detection of unanticipated changes in the protection program. For facilities that have low workloads, a three-month replacement interval is a good compromise. Personal dosimeters using film, however, are inaccurate when used for periods longer than one month.

C.4 Conclusion

Dental radiation protection programs may range in complexity and effort from very simple, such as that of a private office, to fairly sophisticated, such as that of a dental school. While larger facilities often have access to radiation protection expertise and equipment, and hence provide more formal radiation protection programs, private office community based facilities also need to have a radiation protection program. A small investment of time and effort by the individual practitioner can result in lower radiation risks to patients and an improved work environment for staff members.

Appendix D

Selection Criteria

Selection criteria are those historical and clinical findings that suggest that radiographs are likely to contribute diagnostic information useful for proper care of the patient. The need for an x-ray examination, the type of examination indicated, and the potential that the examination may be beneficial to the patient can be determined only by the professional judgment of the dentist. It is imperative that x-ray exposure of a patient be done only on the basis of patient history, physical examination, or laboratory findings. Common examples of history and physical findings suggesting the need for radiographs are clinical signs of periodontitis, caries, large restorations including crowns, and a history of endodontic therapy. As the individual circumstances of each patient will vary, so will the need for radiographs. No routine time-based formula for obtaining radiographs will be applicable to all patients in a dental practice. Thus, judgments made for the care of a specific patient, including radiographic examination, can be made only by using training and experience to integrate data into a comprehensive understanding of that patient's needs.

A guide to selection criteria for dental x-ray examinations of asymptomatic patients (Table D.1) has been developed (Joseph, 1987). It is a useful adjunct for decisions regarding some radiographic examinations. These guidelines, endorsed by the American Dental Association (ADA, 1989), recommend the use of "selected periapicals," that is, the use of individual periapical radiographs selected by a dentist to examine a specific tooth or region because of specific signs, symptoms, or historical findings that suggest a high likelihood of findings that will influence patient management (Joseph, 1987). Bitewing examinations are recommended on a periodic basis depending on the age and oral health of the patient. There is insufficient evidence of diagnostic yield to warrant periodic radiographic examination of all the tooth-bearing regions in search of occult pathology in the asymptomatic dental patient. Several studies have documented the efficacy of using selection criteria in dentistry (Brooks, 1986; Brooks and Cho, 1993; Matteson *et al.*, 1983). Clinical validation of these guidelines in a dental school clinic population showed that use of these guidelines resulted in a 44 percent reduction in the number of periapical radiographs ordered without a clinically significant increase in the rate of missed disease (Atchison *et al.*, 1995). Other evidence suggests that there is little or no diagnostic benefit to obtaining a panoramic examination and a simultaneous full-mouth set of radiographs for the purpose of general patient screening (Joseph, 1987). In this situation the panoramic is unlikely to offer clinically significant new information.

The recommendations in Table D.1 can be used for pregnant patients, with the further caveat that special care should be taken to minimize exposure to the embryo or fetus.

TABLE D.1—*Selection criteria for dental radiographic examinations in asymptomatic patients.*[a]

Patient Category	Child		Adolescent	Adult	
	Primary Dentition (prior to eruption of first permanent tooth)	Transitional Dentition (following eruption of first permanent tooth)	Permanent Dentition (prior to eruption of third molars)	Dentulous	Edentulous
NEW PATIENT All new patients to assess dental diseases and growth and development	Posterior bitewing examination if proximal surfaces of primary teeth cannot be visualized or probed	Individualized radiographic examination consisting of periapical or occlusal views and posterior bitewings or panoramic examination and posterior bitewings	Individualized radiographic examination consisting of posterior bitewings and selected periapicals. A full mouth intraoral radiographic examination is appropriate when the patient presents with clinical evidence of generalized dental disease or a history of extensive dental treatment		Full mouth intraoral radiographic examination or panoramic examination
RECALL PATIENT[b] Clinical caries or high-risk factors for caries[c]	Posterior bitewing examination at six month intervals or until no carious lesions are evident		Posterior bitewing examinations at 6 to 12 month intervals or until no carious lesions are evident	Posterior bitewing examination at 12 to 18 month intervals	Not applicable

RECALL PATIENT[b] No clinical caries and no high-risk factors for caries[c]	Posterior bitewing examination at 12 to 24 month intervals if proximal surfaces of primary teeth cannot be visualized or probed	Posterior bitewing examinations at 12 to 24 month intervals	Posterior bitewing examinations at 12 to 24 month intervals	Posterior bitewing examinations at 24 to 36 month intervals	Not applicable
RECALL PATIENT[b] Periodontal disease or a history of periodontal involvement	Individualized radiographic examination consisting of selected periapical and/or bitewing radiographs for areas where periodontal disease (other than nonspecific gingivitis) can be demonstrated clinically		Individualized radiographic examination consisting of selected periapical and/or bitewing radiographs for areas where periodontal disease (other than nonspecific gingivitis) can be demonstrated clinically		Not applicable
RECALL PATIENT[b] Growth and development assessment	Usually not indicated	Individualized radiographic examination consisting of a periapical/occlusal or panoramic examination	Periapical or panoramic examination to assess developing third molars	Usually not indicated	Usually not indicated

[a]The recommendations in this table are subject to clinical judgment and may not apply to every patient. They are to be used by dentists only after reviewing the patient's health history and completing a clinical examination (data from Joseph, 1987).

[b]Clinical situations for which radiographs may be indicated include:

A. Positive historical findings
   1. Previous periodontal or endodontic therapy
   2. Pain or trauma
   3. Family history of dental anomalies
   4. Postoperative evaluation of healing
   5. Presence of implants

B. Positive clinical signs/symptoms
   1. Evidence of periodontal disease
   2. Large or deep restorations
   3. Deep carious lesions
   4. Malposed or impacted teeth
   5. Swelling
   6. Evidence of facial trauma
   7. Mobility of teeth
   8. Fistula or sinus tract infection
   9. Suspected sinus pathology
   10. Growth abnormalities
   11. Oral involvement in known or suspected systemic disease
   12. Positive neurologic findings in the head and neck
   13. Evidence of foreign objects
   14. Pain and/or dysfunction of temporomandibular joint
   15. Facial asymmetry
   16. Abutment teeth for fixed or removable partial prosthesis
   17. Unexplained bleeding
   18. Unexplained sensitivity of teeth
   19. Unusual eruption, spacing, or migration of teeth
   20. Unusual tooth morphology, calcification or color
   21. Missing teeth with unknown reason

[c]Patients at high risk for caries may demonstrate any of the following:

1. High level of caries experience
2. History of recurrent caries
3. Existing restoration of poor quality
4. Poor oral hygiene
5. Inadequate fluoride exposure
6. Prolonged nursing (bottle or breast)
7. Diet with high sucrose frequency
8. Poor family dental health
9. Developmental enamel defects
10. Developmental disability
11. Xerostomia
12. Genetic abnormality of teeth
13. Many multisurface restorations
14. Chemo/radiation therapy

Appendix E

Image Receptors

E.1 Characteristics

The performance of image receptor systems can be characterized by five measures: speed, contrast, latitude, resolution and noise. These terms are defined in the Glossary.

E.2 Intraoral Film

Conventional intraoral film is direct exposure film, in that the latent image is produced by the direct exposure of film emulsion by the x-ray beam. Intraoral film is designated by speed groups C through F (ADA, 1970; ANSI, 1996) (Table E.1). Speed groups D, E and F are available for use in intraoral radiography (Farman and Farman, 2000; Thunthy, 2000). Adjacent groups differ in speed by factors of approximately two. Thus, speed group E is approximately twice the speed of group D, *i.e.*, E-speed films permit patient exposure to be reduced by about half of that required for D-speed films (Ludlow and Platin, 1995; Price, 1995). Speed group F is approximately twice the speed of group E.

TABLE E.1—*Intraoral film-speed classification.*[a]

Film-Speed Group	Speed Range (R^{-1})[a]
C	6 – 12
D	12 – 24
E	24 – 48
F	48 – 96

[a]Data from American Dental Association (ADA, 1970), given in the quantity utilized at the time of publication [inverse of exposure in roentgen (R^{-1})].

The introduction of faster film speeds does not result in decreased image quality or diagnostic yield due to alterations in film emulsion. Early group-E film with conventional emulsion technology had a useful density range similar to group-D film, but demonstrated a slight decrease in contrast and was more sensitive to processing conditions (Diehl *et al.*, 1986; Thunthy and Weinberg, 1982). In clinical trials, however, group-E and group-D film demonstrated comparable diagnostic quality (Frommer and Jain, 1987; Kleier *et al.*, 1987; White and Pharaoh, 2004).

A newer type of group-E film employs a new grain technology also employed in screen-film emulsions. In comparative studies, this new group-E film displayed similar contrast to group-D film and less variability under differing processing conditions than the initial group-E film types (Ludlow and Platin, 1995; Price, 1995). Patient exposure can be significantly reduced by utilization of E-speed or F-speed film without compromising diagnostic quality. Further developments in emulsion technology may result in future improvements.

E.3 Screen Films and Intensifying Screens

Extraoral exposures, such as for panoramic and cephalometric radiography, utilize light-sensitive film in combination with intensifying screens within a cassette. The intensifying screens consist of thin layers of phosphor crystals that fluoresce when exposed to x rays. The film is exposed by light emitted by the intensifying screens. Absorption of light emitted from the intensifying screens is increased by the addition of dyes to the film emulsion. The spectrum of light most readily absorbed by the film is matched to the spectrum of light emitted by the intensifying screens. Direct exposure film, such as intraoral films, are relatively insensitive to visible light and intensifying screens do not provide for decreased exposure with these films.

Screen films are widely available with varying speed, contrast and latitude characteristics, depending on specific imaging needs. Screen-film combinations are more sensitive to x rays than nonscreen film, thus reducing the level of exposure to the patient. Image sharpness, however, is decreased as a result of diffusion of light emitted from the intensifying screens to expose the film.

Rare-earth intensifying screens, used in conjunction with properly matched screen films, are the fastest screen-film combinations available as of the date of this Report. Rare-earth screens that emit green or blue light are more efficient at absorbing radiation that exits the patient and converting x-ray energy to light energy than the blue-emitting calcium tungstate screens. Patient exposure in panoramic and cephalometric radiography may be reduced by about 50 percent using fast rare-earth versus slower calcium tungstate screen-film combinations with no significant difference in perceived diagnostic quality (Gratt *et al.*, 1984; Kaugars and Fatouros, 1982). Use of screen film with new grain technology results in increased film speed without a loss of image sharpness. Rare-earth imaging systems using this film have been shown to be 1.3 times faster than a comparable system using conventional film emulsion technology without compromising diagnostic quality (D'Ambrosio *et al.*, 1986; Thunthy and Weinberg, 1986; White and Pharaoh, 2004).

E.4 Direct Digital Radiography

Digital radiography involves the replacement of a film-based image by a digital image consisting of a two-dimensional array of pixels. In direct digital radiography, the latent image is directly recorded by a suitable sensor. Receptors used in direct digital radiography are photostimulable storage phosphor plates or solid state electronic devices containing either charge-coupled device (CCD) or complementary metal-oxide semiconductor technology. In indirect digital radiography, the image is initially recorded on conventional film, and later digitally processed to produce an electronic image. The electronic image may be displayed on a computer monitor, converted to a hard copy, or transmitted electronically.

E.4.1 *Charge-Coupled Device Arrays*

The more common intraoral digital receptor is a two-dimensional CCD array that is connected by cable to a computer. Most CCDs are made of pure silicon and are sensitive to x rays or visible light. The CCD receptor is either directly exposed to x rays or x-ray energy is converted by an intensifying screen to light that is transmitted to the CCD array. An electronic charge, proportional to the amount of x-ray exposure, is accumulated in the CCD. For intraoral projections, the image receptor is positioned intraorally and exposed using conventional techniques. On completion of exposure, the image is immediately digitized and displayed on a computer monitor as well as stored in memory.

E.4.2 *Photostimuable Storage Phosphor Receptors*

The photostimulable storage phosphor plate is similar to an intensifying screen. It is inserted in a light-tight cassette and exposed using conventional techniques (Wenzel and Grondahl, 1995). When the plate is exposed, it does not immediately emit visible light on exposure to radiation. Instead, it stores the latent image in a quasi-stable state. The cassette containing the exposed plate is placed in a processor that removes the plate and positions it on a stage so it can be scanned by a laser, which stimulates photoluminescent emission of the image that can be recorded digitally or transferred to a film (Bushberg *et al.*, 2001). The imaging plates are reusable.

E.4.3 *Features of Direct Digital Radiography*

There are several advantages of direct digital radiography. The image may be rapidly acquired and, in the case of CCD receptors, displayed immediately. There is no darkroom requirement. The image may be electronically manipulated to enhance the perception of certain features; however, there is no increase in diagnostic information content. Images are easily stored and transmitted in digital form. Patient dose may be less than with conventional film (Dunn and Kantor, 1993; Wenzel and Grondahl, 1995). Sensitivity of digital receptors to x radiation may result in exposure reductions greater than 50 percent compared to E-speed film. In many systems, however, the active area of the receptor is smaller than conventional film. Thus, more exposures may be required to image a specified region. In addition, most CCD receptors are thicker than conventional film, which may make intraoral positioning difficult and result in more retakes.

Image resolution is decreased in digital images compared with conventional film. Spatial resolution for direct digital systems ranges from 6 to 10 lp mm^{-1} (line pairs per millimeter) compared to 12 to 14 lp mm^{-1} for radiographic film (Dunn and Kantor, 1993; Wenzel and Grondahl, 1995). Most current direct digital systems provide 256 shades of gray; however, contrast resolution is limited by many computer monitors that can only display 64 shades of gray simultaneously (Wenzel and Grondahl, 1995). Nevertheless, comparative studies have shown that the diagnostic quality of direct digital images approaches that of conventional film in detecting occlusal and approximal caries, periodontal bone lesions, periapical bone lesions and root canal systems (Furkart *et al.*, 1992; Hintze *et al.*, 1994; Kullendorf *et al.*, 1996; Sanderink *et al.*, 1994; Shearer *et al.*, 1990; Svanaes *et al.*, 1996).

Appendix F

Shielding Design for Dental Facilities

An NCRP report entitled, *Structural Shielding Design for Medical X-Ray Imaging Facilities* (NCRP, in press), will discuss concepts and examples of shielding design for x-ray sources with operating potentials in the range from 25 to 150 kVp (kilovolt peak) (see Glossary). Techniques used for calculating shielding barriers for diagnostic medical x-rays also have been discussed in the literature (Dixon and Simpkin, 1998; Simpkin and Dixon, 1998). Since dental radiography uses equipment similar in radiation quality to that used in diagnostic medical x-ray facilities, much of the following discussion is drawn from those sources.

Conventional building materials in partitions, floors and ceilings may provide adequate radiation shielding for dental installations. However, any assumption of the adequacy of conventional barriers can lead to a false sense of security.

F.1 General Principles

An x-ray tube in a dental radiology facility provides three sources of x radiation, each of which requires analysis for radiation shielding requirements. These are primary, scattered and leakage radiation.

Primary radiation is that generated in the anode of the x-ray tube, emanating from the x-ray tube portal, and directed toward the patient and image receptor. The energies of the primary photons range from approximately 15 keV (kiloelectron volt) to an energy in keV numerically equal to the maximal x-ray tube operating potential. This potential is determined by the demands of radiographic contrast, but typically ranges from 60 to 90 kVp for intraoral dental radiography. Recently manufactured dental radiography units do not exceed 100 kVp. The dose rate from primary radiation is dependent on the operating potential (kVp), proportional to the x-ray tube current (milliamperes), and inversely proportional to the square of the distance from the x-ray tube focal spot to the occupied area (i.e., follows the inverse square law).

Scattered radiation is created by Compton and coherent interactions in objects struck by the primary photons, particularly the patient. Scattered radiation is an unavoidable consequence of the primary beam. The air-kerma rate due to scattered radiation is proportional to the primary beam air-kerma rate and the angular breadth of the primary beam, and inversely proportional to the square of the distance from the scattering medium to the occupied area. The direction of the scattered x rays is fairly random, with some preference to backscattering. While the scattered photon energy spectrum is shifted to lower energies as a result of Compton interactions, for radiation protection purposes, the scattered radiation spectrum may be assumed to match that of the primary beam.

Leakage radiation is generated in the x-ray tube anode and is transmitted through the protective housing. This hardens the transmitted radiation to the point that only the most energetic photons are assumed to constitute leakage radiation. The air-kerma rate due to leakage radiation generated under particular conditions is limited by regulation. When the x-ray tube is operated at its leakage technique factors, the leakage radiation at 1 m from the source is limited to an exposure rate of 0.1 R h^{-1} (equivalent to an air-kerma rate of 0.876 mGy h^{-1}) by the U.S. standard (FDA, 1995). The international leakage radiation standard is an air-kerma rate of 0.25 mGy h^{-1} for intraoral machines and 1 mGy h^{-1} for all other machines (IEC, 1994). Most recently produced equipment is manufactured to meet the international standard, to be able to market the equipment on a worldwide basis. The emission of leakage photons is assumed to be randomly directed from the x-ray tube. Scattered and leakage radiation are said to be secondary radiation.

The primary, scattered, and leakage radiation therefore differ in their intensity, point of origin, and photon energy distribution. Due to these differences, they also differ in transmission through a barrier. The total air kerma[4] transmitted to an occupied area [$K_{tot}(x,\mathrm{m})$] due to radiation from an x-ray tube in a radiologic room, shielded by a barrier of thickness x of material m, is the sum of the

[4]In this Report, the symbol K always refers to the quantity air kerma (in place of the usual symbol K_a), followed by an appropriate subscript to further describe the quantity (*e.g.*, K_P, air kerma from primary radiation).

primary, scattered and leakage air-kerma contributions from the tube. Thus if $K_P(x,\text{m})$, $K_S(x,\text{m})$, and $K_L(x,\text{m})$ are the air kerma transmitted to the occupied area from primary, scattered and leakage radiation respectively, then:

$$K_{tot}(x,\text{m}) = K_P(x,\text{m}) + K_S(x,\text{m}) + K_L(x,\text{m}). \tag{F.1}$$

If a room contains more than one x-ray tube, the contributions from each tube need to be summed.

A radiation barrier of thickness x_{acc} is deemed acceptable when the total air kerma at a point beyond the barrier (usually assumed to be 0.3 m) is equal to or less than the appropriate shielding design goal (*i.e.*, 0.1 mGy week^{-1} for controlled areas and 0.02 mGy week^{-1} for uncontrolled areas) (NCRP, in press). These weekly shielding design goals correspond to annual air-kerma values of 5 mGy (controlled areas) and 1 mGy (uncontrolled areas) (NCRP, in press).

Shielding design goals for dental x-ray sources are practical values that result in the respective limits for effective dose in a year to workers and the public not being exceeded, when combined with conservatively safe assumptions in the structural shielding design calculations (NCRP, in press). Additionally, the shielding design goal is expressed as a weekly value since workload, occupancy factor, and other technical data needed for structural shielding calculations of facilities utilize a weekly format.

Controlled areas are those where employees have significant potential for exposure to radiation in the course of their assignments, or where the employees are directly responsible for or involved with the use and control of radiation. These individuals generally have training in radiation management and are subject to routine personal monitoring. Uncontrolled areas are those occupied by individuals such as patients, visitors to the facility, and employees who do not work routinely with or around radiation sources. Areas adjacent to but not part of the x-ray facility are also uncontrolled areas.

For cases where an individual only occupies the shielded area a fraction T of the time (T is the "occupancy factor"), the shielding design goal P is adjusted by the factor T^{-1}. Therefore, an acceptable radiation-shielding barrier is defined by:

$$K_{tot}(x_{acc}, \text{m}) = \frac{P}{T}\ . \tag{F.2}$$

In general, the acceptable barrier thickness x_{acc} can be determined from Equation F.2 only by using numerical or graphical methods. That is, the total air kerma through a barrier of thickness x is calculated from Equation F.1 utilizing the models for the primary, scattered, and leakage air kerma (Appendix F.3), and modified until Equation F.2 is satisfied. For some cases, x_{acc} can be determined approximately using tables developed for simplified conditions. Examples of simplified calculations are given in Appendix F.4.

F.2 Barrier Thickness Calculations

The equations given in Appendix F.3 may be used to solve for the exact barrier thickness required to achieve the appropriate value of *P*. Their use is indicated for circumstances in which the radiation quality and exposure level are accurately known and optimal (least thickness) shielding is desired. In other circumstances a less precise, simpler to implement and more conservatively safe (*i.e.*, barrier thickness may be overestimated) approach may be applied using the "table method" discussed in Appendix F.5.

To estimate *a priori* the air kerma in an occupied area beyond the barrier due to primary, scattered and leakage radiation, assumptions need to be made of the room's layout, the magnitude of the x-ray tube use, and the efficiency with which a barrier attenuates the photons from that tube. Estimates of the distances from the x-ray tube and the patient to the occupied locations should be accurate and conservatively short. Figure F.1 shows a hypothetical dental x-ray imaging room, in which only one intraoral x-ray machine serves one patient.

F.2.1 *Determining Protective Barrier Requirements*

Numerical values for a number of variables are needed to compute a barrier thickness. These variables are:

- the maximum operating potential (maximum kVp) of the x-ray machine used for radiography
- the workload of the x-ray tube in units of milliampere-minutes per week
- the distance to the point of calculation for primary or secondary barriers (as shown in Figures F.2 and F.3)
- the weekly shielding design goal for a controlled or uncontrolled area

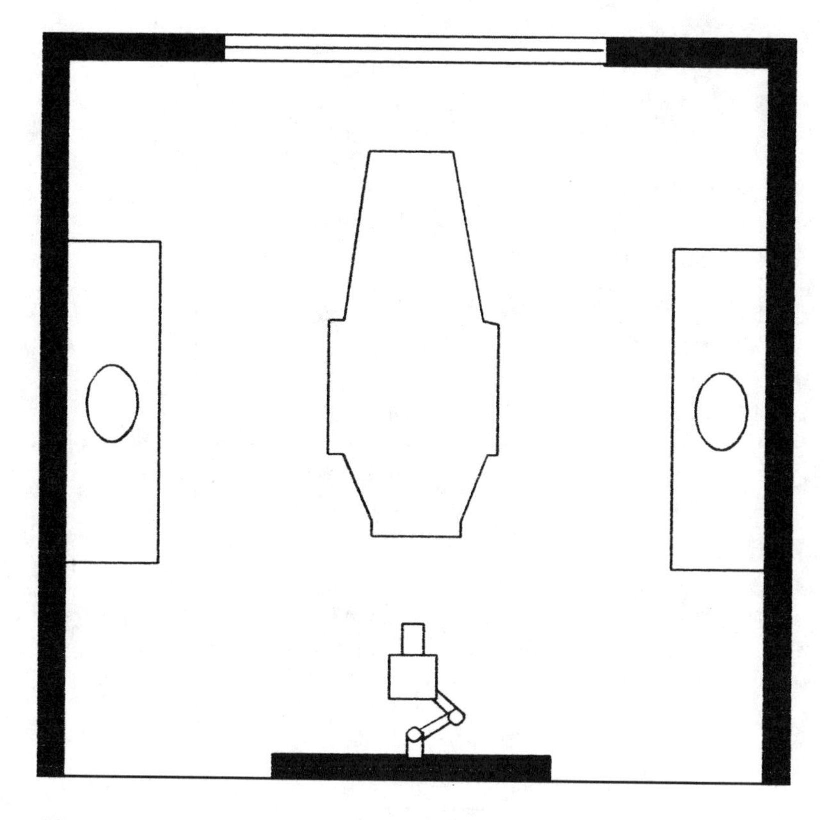

Fig. F.1. Typical layout of an intraoral radiography and dental procedure room in which one x-ray unit is dedicated to one patient (Malkin, 2002).

- the fraction of the total "ON" time of the x-ray tube during which a person is in the vicinity of the radiation source in an uncontrolled area (occupancy factor, see Table F.1); for a controlled area the occupancy factor is one
- the fraction of the total "ON" time the x-ray tube is directed toward a primary barrier (use factor, see Table F.2)
- the fraction of primary beam transmitted through the patient and image receptor (measured or see Figure F.4)
- the leakage radiation standard to which the tube was designed and the effective leakage current.

F.2.1.1 *Operating Potential (Kilovolt Peak).* The operating potential of the x-ray tube, expressed as kilovolt peak (kVp, see Glossary), needs to be known to account for the x-ray energy

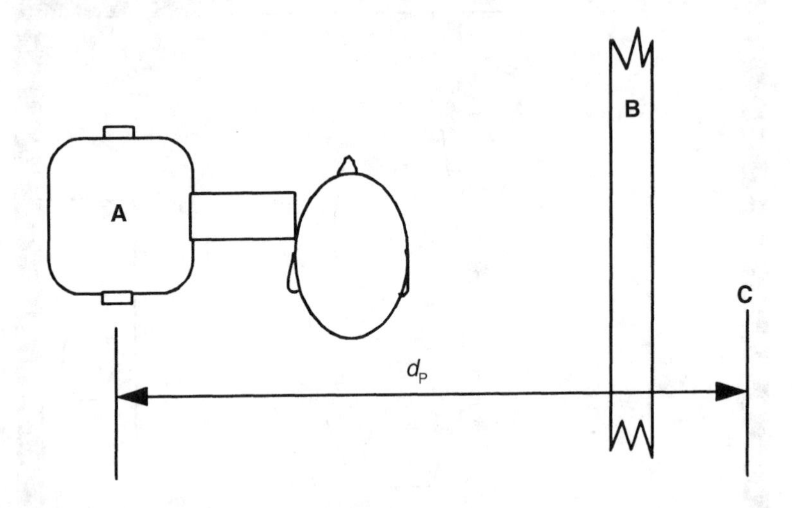

Fig. F.2. Diagram illustrating primary barrier B, protecting person at C from useful beam at a distance d_P from dental x ray source A.

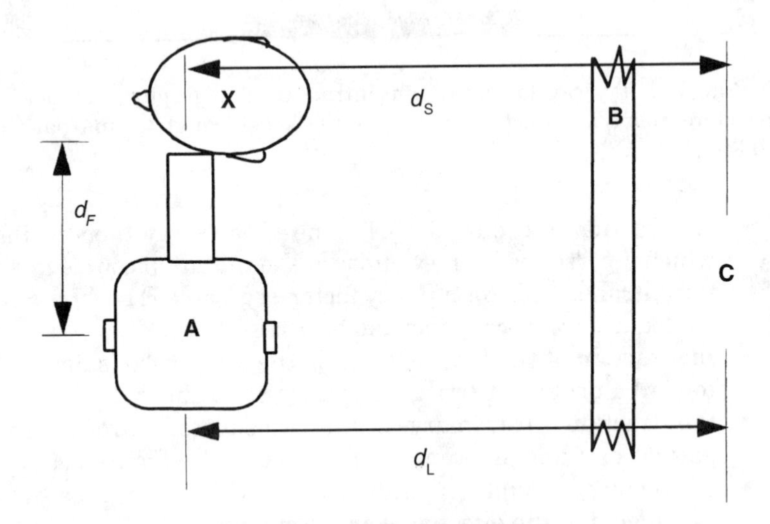

Fig. F.3. Diagram illustrating secondary barrier B, protecting a person at C from scattered radiation from patient X at a distance d_S and from leakage radiation from x ray tube housing A at a distance d_L. F is the primary field size at a distance d_F from the primary source.

TABLE F.1—*Suggested occupancy factors*[a] *(for use as a guide in planning shielding where other occupancy data are not available) (NCRP, in press).*

Location	Occupancy Factor (T)
Administrative or clerical offices; laboratories, pharmacies and other work areas fully occupied by an individual; receptionist area, attended waiting rooms, children's indoor play areas, adjacent x-ray rooms, film reading area, nurse's stations, x-ray control rooms	1
Patient examination and treatment rooms	1/2
Corridors, patient rooms, employee lounges, staff toilets	1/5
Public toilets, unattended vending areas, storage rooms, outer areas with seating, unattended waiting rooms, patient holding areas	1/20
Outdoor areas with only transient pedestrian or vehicular traffic, unattended parking lots, vehicular drop off areas (unattended), attics, stairways, unattended elevators, janitor's closets	1/40

[a]When using a low occupancy factor for a room immediately adjacent to an x-ray room, care should be taken to also consider the areas further removed from the x-ray room that may have significantly higher occupancy factors and may therefore be more important in shielding design despite the larger distances involved.

TABLE F.2—*Suggested use factors for intraoral radiography units (MacDonald et al., 1983; Reid and MacDonald, 1984).*

Barrier	Use Factor (U)
Side walls	0.4
Back wall (wall facing patient's back)	0.2
Front wall (wall facing patient's front)	0
Ceiling	0
Floor	0

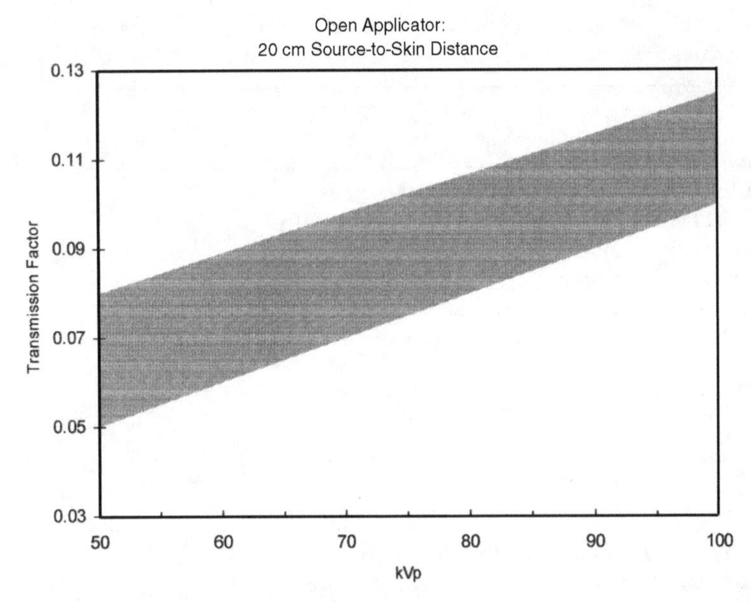

Fig. F.4. Measured transmission through a typical patient of primary dental x rays from right and left bitewing exposures. The range of transmission factors at a given kVp reflects the range of typical tissue thickness (MacDonald *et al.*, 1983).

dependence of barrier transmission. The amount of leakage radiation also depends upon kVp. A conservatively safe calculation assumes that the unit always is operated at its maximum value of kVp. However, if clinical use dictates that a unit is consistently operated at a kVp (or range of kVp) below the maximum, the actual clinical kVp may be used.

F.2.1.2 *Workload.* The magnitude of the x-ray tube use is stated as the tube workload. The transmission is the fraction by which the air kerma is decreased due to the presence of the shielding barrier. The workload and transmission are typically strong functions of the tube operating potential. The workload of an x-ray tube is the product of the x-ray tube current and the time for which the x-ray tube is operating at that current. The unit for the workload is milliampere-second (mAs) or milliampere-minute (mA min), usually stated per week of x-ray tube operation. The workload is a direct measure of the number of electrons incident on the x-ray tube anode. At a given operating potential, workload is directly proportional to the air kerma in the primary beam at a specified distance. Calculations are considerably simpler if it is assumed that the x-ray tube only operates at a single potential. For many situations in dental radiography, particularly intraoral radiography, this is a good assumption. If a range of operating potential is used, calculations may be performed in a conservatively safe manner by assuming all the workload is at the highest used operating potential.

The workload for diagnostic shielding calculations is expressed in milliampere-minutes per week (mA min $week^{-1}$), which is the product of x-ray tube current and exposure time summed over a one-week interval. Workload may be converted to air kerma, in units of milligray per week, by multiplying by the air kerma per unit workload at 1 m, in units of mGy mA^{-1} min^{-1}. As discussed below, the air kerma per unit workload is dependent on kVp and waveform, and increases approximately as the square of the kVp. For comparable film optical density, less milliampere-seconds are required for higher kVp, and the total air kerma produced per week is approximately independent of kVp. However, knowledge of the kVp is still necessary, since the barrier transmission and head leakage depend strongly on kVp.

Waveform of an x-ray machine refers to the temporal variation of the operating potential applied to the x-ray tube during the course of an exposure. Most dental x-ray machines are single-phase, half-wave rectified. In these machines, x rays are produced only during half of each 1/60 s alternating current cycle. During that half-cycle, voltage across the x-ray tube goes from zero to the kVp and back to zero in a hemi-sinusoidal wave; it remains at zero during the second half-cycle as the line voltage reverses. The x-ray beam energy ranges during this half-cycle from no emission to a maximum equal to the kVp and back to no emission. Average photon energy (in keV) is substantially less than (generally less than half) the kVp value. Some newer machines approach constant potential from single-phase current, in which tube voltage is electronically manipulated to remain at or near the kVp throughout the exposure. From these machines, average photon energy (in keV) is a much greater fraction of the kVp value. Some medical but few dental machines use three-phase current with voltage inversion, such that there are 12 overlapping voltage pulses during each 1/60 s cycle, producing a mean tube voltage approaching that of the kVp.

Workload also depends on cone length. For the same image receptor, the required milliampere-seconds for a 40 cm cone is four times that of a 20 cm cone. Studies of exposure patterns on the walls of dental radiography suites have shown that use of long cones does not result in four times greater barrier exposure (Reid and MacDonald, 1984). This is due to greater overlap of radiation distributions with the short, more divergent, cone. Reid and MacDonald (1984) have proposed that the number of films per week, rather than the total milliampere-seconds per week, is a more representative measure of workload. In this Report however, it is a conservatively safe assumption that workload is calculated only from milliampere-minutes per week, ignoring possible ameliorating effects of less overlap with less divergent cones.

Workload, expressed in milliampere-minutes per week, can be determined by counting the number of films exposed over several weeks and averaging the number for each week. The product of the average number of films per week and the average milliampere-seconds per film divided by 60 (to convert milliampere-seconds to milliampere-minutes) will yield the workload in milliampere-minutes per week. Workload for other types of dental imaging is determined in the same manner, by multiplying examinations per week times the average milliampere times the exposure time in seconds and dividing by 60. Table F.3 can be used to estimate the typical workload of dental units if detailed information is not available.

F.2.1.3 *Use Factor.* The fraction of the x-ray emission time during which the x-ray beam is pointed toward a specific barrier is termed the use factor for that barrier. Suggested values for use factors given in Table F.2 may be used if specific values are not known.

F.2.1.3.1 *Intraoral radiography.* In intraoral radiography, as shown in Figure F.5, when the patient is facing wall J, the useful beam could strike either the walls G, H and I, but not the wall J (the wall the patient faces). The floor and ceiling are rarely, if ever struck by the primary beam. Use factors and distribution of radiation exposure on the walls of intraoral facilities have been investigated (MacDonald *et al.*, 1983; Reid and MacDonald, 1984). These studies suggest that the use factor for lateral walls (G and I) should be 0.4, and for posterior wall H should be 0.2. The use factor for anterior wall J and the floor and ceiling is zero. Although collimated to small field sizes at the patient, the radiation fields do overlap at the walls. Due to the greater divergence, overlap is greater with short cones as compared to long cones (Reid and MacDonald, 1984).

A popular technique for intraoral radiography using positive beam-alignment (Section 3.1.4.1.3) consists of reclining the patient and achieving desired geometry by rotating the patients head, while maintaining the primary beam at or near vertical (aimed at

TABLE F.3—*Estimated workload for intraoral and panoramic units.*[a,b]

Type of Unit	Total Films or Images per Week per Unit	kVp	mAs per Film or Image	Film Speed or Image Receptor Speed	Workload (mA min $week^{-1}$)
Low volume intraoral	100	50	8.5	E	14
		70	4.5		7.5
		90	2.5		4.2
Medium volume intraoral	200	50	8.5	E	28
		70	4.5		15
		90	2.5		8.3
High volume intraoral	300	50	8.5	E	43
		70	4.5		23
		90	2.5		13
Low volume panoramic	25	50	180	400	75
		70	100		42
		90	60		25
Medium volume panoramic	50	50	180	400	150
		70	100		83
		90	60		50
High volume panoramic	75	50	180	400	225
		70	100		125
		90	60		75

[a]The intraoral workload assumes a single-phase waveform and that a 40 cm cone is used. If image receptors having a speed different from those given in Table F.3 are used, the workload should be scaled by the ratio of the film or image receptor speeds. For instance, workload should be doubled for D-speed film. For a constant-potential waveform, the technique factor (milliampere-seconds) and workload should be reduced by about one-third.

[b]In the absence of other specific local data, the entries in this Table are suggested in this Report.

the floor). When this technique is used, the floor becomes a primary barrier and cannot be neglected.

Intraoral radiography is performed with the beam tightly collimated to the patient's head. In addition, a lead foil backed film packet covers a significant fraction of the collimated radiation field. The combination of patient and image receptor significantly

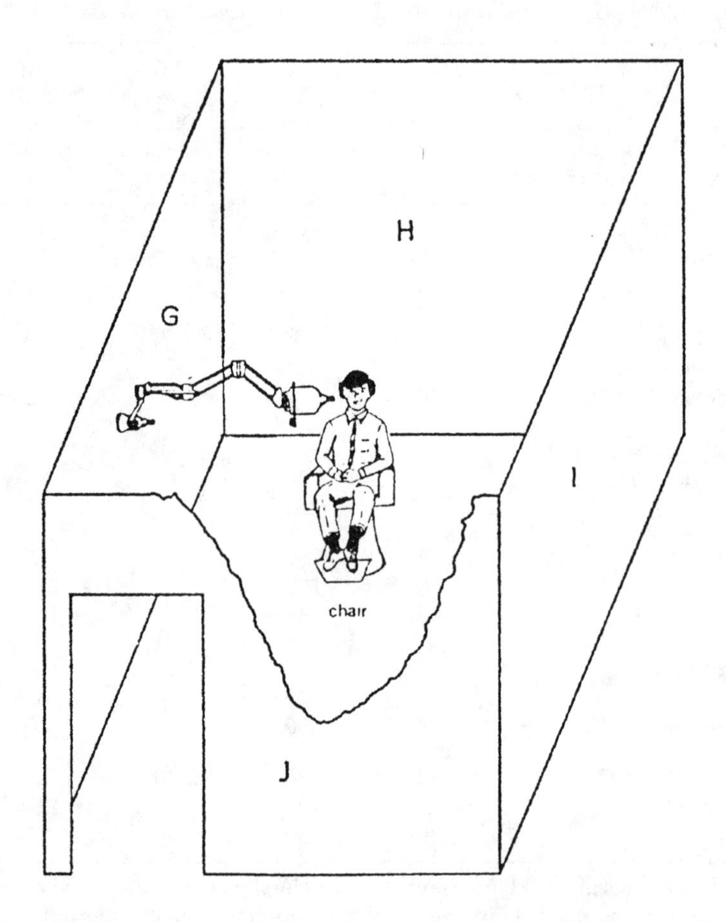

Fig. F.5. View of a dental x-ray installation during the exposure of intraoral films. The useful beam might strike walls G, H and I. All of the walls, the ceiling, and the floor are likely to be struck by scattered radiation (NCRP, 1970).

attenuates the primary radiation. MacDonald *et al.* (1983) measured patient transmission factors of 0.05 to 0.125, over the range of 50 to 100 kVp (Figure F.4). When combined with a use factor of 0.4, a patient attenuation factor of 0.1 results in an effective use factor of about 0.04. NCRP Report No. 35 (NCRP, 1970) recommended a use factor of 1/16 (0.0625) to account for both effects. In this Report, patient attenuation effects are considered explicitly (see discussion of a_{pt} in Appendix F.3.1), and the use factor accounts only for the fraction of the x-ray emission time during which the x-ray beam is pointed towards a specific barrier.

F.2.1.3.2 *Panoramic radiography.* Panoramic machines have a narrow, slit-like useful beam that irradiates a relatively small portion of the head at any one time. The amount of scattered radiation from the patient is relatively less than that in multiple periapical (full mouth) examinations. Furthermore, the direction of the beam in a panoramic machine is fixed to strike the aperture on the image-receptor holding device that has a primary barrier behind the image receptor. The useful beam traverses only the patient area to be examined and does not strike other objects. In the case of panoramic machines then, only secondary barriers are required. Reid *et al.* (1993) measured the air- kerma levels around a panoramic machine whose maximum technique was 90 kVp and 12 mA, but was typically operated at 75 kVp and up to 10 mA. Under those conditions, an average air kerma of 4.5×10^{-5} mGy per exposure was measured and they concluded that no additional shielding was required. The low value of secondary radiation per exposure was due in large part to the machine being operated well below its maximum leakage radiation conditions.

F.2.1.4 *Occupancy Factor.* The occupancy factor is the fraction of time a shielded area is occupied during the time the source may be "ON." Occupancy factors for areas frequented by occupationally-exposed individuals (*i.e.*, controlled areas) are assumed to be unity. If no other information is available, Table F.1 (NCRP, in press) may be used to estimate occupancy factors for persons in uncontrolled areas adjacent to the radiographic room, and allows greater specificity in determining occupancy factors, particularly for low occupancy areas.

F.2.1.5 *X-Ray Leakage Characteristics.* Dental x-ray tube housings are manufactured to meet regulatory standards for leakage radiation. For older equipment and equipment manufactured to meet only the U.S. standard, leakage radiation cannot exceed an exposure rate of 0.1 R h^{-1} (*i.e.*, an air-kerma rate of 0.876 mGy h^{-1}) at 1 m when the tube is operated at its maximum continuous current (FDA, 1995). For equipment manufactured to meet international standards, leakage radiation cannot exceed 0.25 mGy h^{-1} at 1 m when the tube is operated at its "maximum duty cycle" (IEC, 1994). The latter concept recognizes that, while the design of dental x-ray tubes does not allow continuous operation, the maximum integrated current in an hour of operation is limited by the heat capacity of the stationary anode. Thus the duty factor of a dental x-ray tube is the fraction of an hour that the tube can be operated at its maximum instantaneous tube current. For an intraoral tube head designed to operate at a single operating potential of 70 kVp and a single (maximum) tube current of 7 mA, the duty factor is typically about 1/30 (Molteni, 1999).[5] Since the formalism of leakage calculation assumes a continuous current, an effective continuous leakage current may be calculated as the product of maximum tube current and duty factor. For the case mentioned above, the effective continuous leakage current is 0.23 mA (*i.e.*, 7/30). Tube heads designed for panoramic radiography often differ from intraoral heads, and may typically shield leakage radiation at a leakage technique of 100 kVp, 15 mA and a duty factor of 1/20 (Molteni, 1999).[5]

F.2.2 *Shielding Design Goals*

Table 1.1 (Section 1.3) gives the annual effective dose limits for occupational and public exposures. For shielding design purposes, however, the ALARA principle (NCRP, 1990) also should be given consideration during the shielding design. For example, for dental x-ray installations, the increased cost in choosing a more restrictive goal for design purposes is usually minimal because of the relatively low x-ray energies used in dental radiography. Shielding design goals (in air kerma) of 0.1 mGy week^{-1} for controlled areas and 0.02 mGy week^{-1} for uncontrolled areas are recommended in NCRP (in press). These shielding design goals are intended for use in planning and designing new facilities and in remodeling existing facilities only. Dental facilities designed before publication of NCRP (in press) and this Report, using the recommendations in NCRP (1970), need not be reevaluated.

F.3 Formalism of Shielding Calculations

The broad beam transmission (B) of x rays through a shielding barrier is defined as the ratio of the air kerma from a wide x-ray beam at a point beyond the barrier in an occupied area when shielded (K_{sh}) to that in an unshielded condition (K_{un}):

[5]Molteni, R. (1999). Personal communication (Gendex Dental X-Ray, DesPlaines Illinois).

$$B = \frac{K_{sh}}{K_{un}} . \tag{F.3}$$

Transmission depends on the type of radiation delivering the air kerma, the energy of the radiation, and the thickness and material constituting the barrier. The scatter transmission is assumed to be equal to that of the primary beam, since to a first approximation the energy spectrum of scattered photons is the same as that for primary photons generated at less than 150 kVp. The transmission of leakage radiation is assumed exponential, since penetration through the tube housing will have removed all but the highest energy x rays generated in the tube. For tube operation at a given potential, the leakage radiation transmission will exceed the primary and scattered radiation transmission. The half-value layer of the leakage radiation is obtained from the primary beam transmission at high attenuation.

Transmission data from the literature will be reviewed and summarized by NCRP (in press). Figures F.6 to F.11 show graphs of the broad-beam transmission of x rays with single-phase waveforms[6] and three-phase or constant-potential waveforms through lead, concrete, gypsum wallboard, steel, plate glass, and wood. The transmission curves have been found to be adequately described by a three-parameter model due to Archer *et al.* (1983). The transmission $B(x,\mathrm{m},V_t)$ through a barrier of thickness x is given by:

$$B(x,\mathrm{m},V_t) = \left\{\left[1 + \frac{\beta(\mathrm{m},V_t)}{\alpha(\mathrm{m},V_t)}\right] e^{\alpha(\mathrm{m},V_t)\gamma(\mathrm{m},V_t)x} - \frac{\beta(\mathrm{m},V_t)}{\alpha(\mathrm{m},V_t)}\right\}^{-\frac{1}{\gamma(\mathrm{m},V_t)}} , \tag{F.4}$$

[6]The x-ray spectrum from single-phase half-wave rectified units is identical to that of full-wave rectified units, therefore, the barrier transmission is the same. Care needs to be taken in the calculation of workload for half-wave rectified units if starting from technique charts. In this Report, workload is given in units of milliampere-minutes per week. Half-wave or self-rectified technique charts use "mAi" (milliampere impulses), the product of the milliamperes and the number of impulses (half waves) used to deliver the exposure. The conversion is given by mA min = mAi/7,200 and does not depend on the time interval between the initiation and termination of exposure. If the "typical" workloads given in this Report in terms of milliampere-minutes per week are used (rather than calculating actual workload from clinical technique charts and actual work volume experience), the conversion above would not be needed.

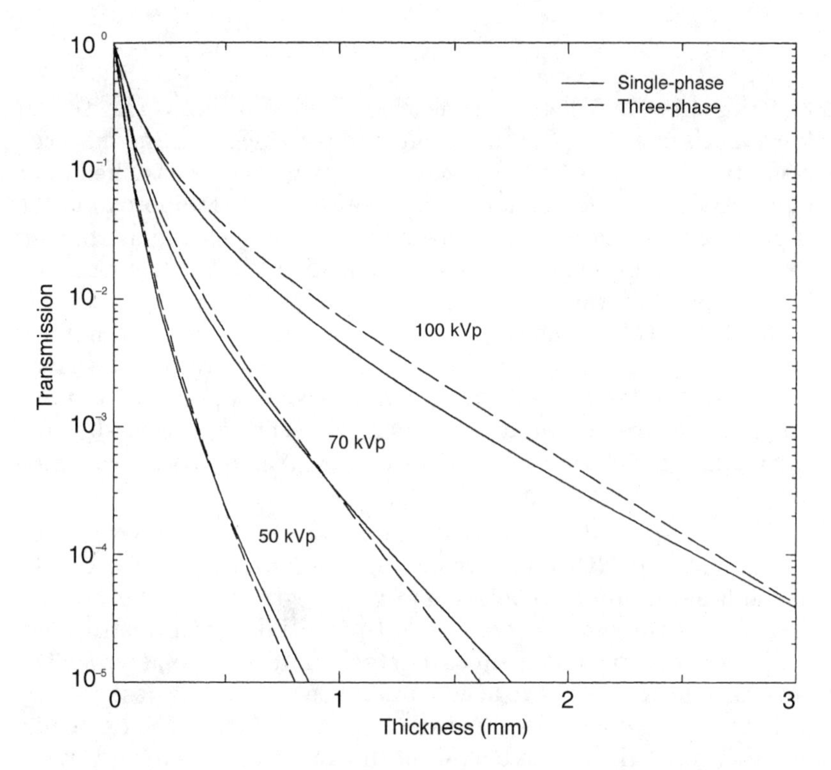

Fig. F.6. Barrier transmission for lead as a function of kVp and waveform (data are plotted from parameters given by Archer *et al.*, 1994). Note that the crossing of the single-phase and three-phase transmission curves for 50 and 70 kVp is the result of curve fitting for data that extended only to a transmission of 10^{-3}. The three-phase transmission curves also apply to constant-potential waveforms.

where the fitting parameters $\alpha(\mathrm{m},V_\mathrm{t})$, $\beta(\mathrm{m},V_\mathrm{t})$ and $\gamma(\mathrm{m},V_\mathrm{t})$ depend on the barrier material m, waveform and the operating potential V_t (*i.e.*, kVp). This can be inverted so that:

$$x(B,\mathrm{m},V_\mathrm{t}) = \frac{1}{\alpha(\mathrm{m},V_\mathrm{t})\ \gamma(\mathrm{m},V_\mathrm{t})} \ln\left[\frac{B^{-\gamma(\mathrm{m},V_\mathrm{t})} + \dfrac{\beta(\mathrm{m},V_\mathrm{t})}{\alpha(\mathrm{m},V_\mathrm{t})}}{1 + \dfrac{\beta(\mathrm{m},V_\mathrm{t})}{\alpha(\mathrm{m},V_\mathrm{t})}}\right]. \qquad \text{(F.5)}$$

For large values of x, known as the high attenuation condition, the transmission curves tend toward an exponential that decreases with constant half-value layer $x_{1/2}(\mathrm{m},V_\mathrm{t})$, given by:

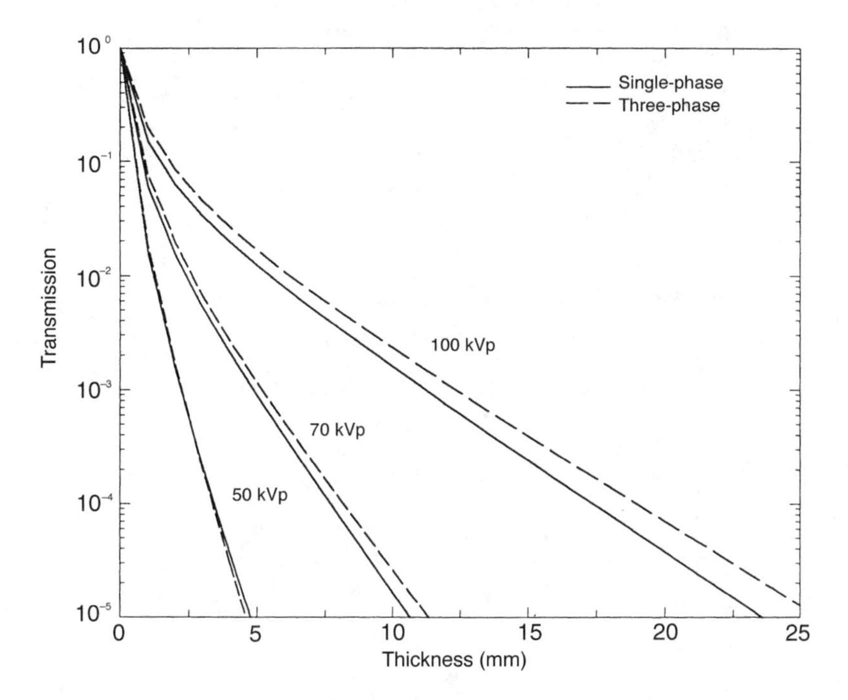

Fig. F.7. Barrier transmission for steel as a function of kVp and waveform (data are plotted from parameters given by Archer *et al.*, 1994). Note that the crossing of the single-phase and three-phase transmission curves for 50 kVp is the result of curve fitting for data that extended only to a transmission of 10^{-3}. The three-phase transmission curves also apply to constant-potential waveforms.

$$x_{1/2}(\mathrm{m},V_\mathrm{t}) = \frac{0.693}{\alpha(\mathrm{m},V_\mathrm{t})} \ . \tag{F.6}$$

Tables F.4a and F.4b give the fitting parameters $\alpha(\mathrm{m},V_\mathrm{t})$, $\beta(\mathrm{m},V_\mathrm{t})$, and $\gamma(\mathrm{m},V_\mathrm{t})$ for the broad beam x-ray transmission of three-phase or constant-potential waveforms (Table F.4a) and single-phase waveforms (Table F.4b) through lead, concrete, gypsum wallboard, steel, plate glass, and wood.

The shielding design goal is given in the quantity air kerma (K), which is routinely measured by ionization chambers. Most literature on shielding is presented in terms of the quantity exposure (X), determined by similar measurements. The air kerma (in milligray) is directly proportional to the exposure (in roentgen), given by:

$$K = 8.76\,X. \tag{F.7}$$

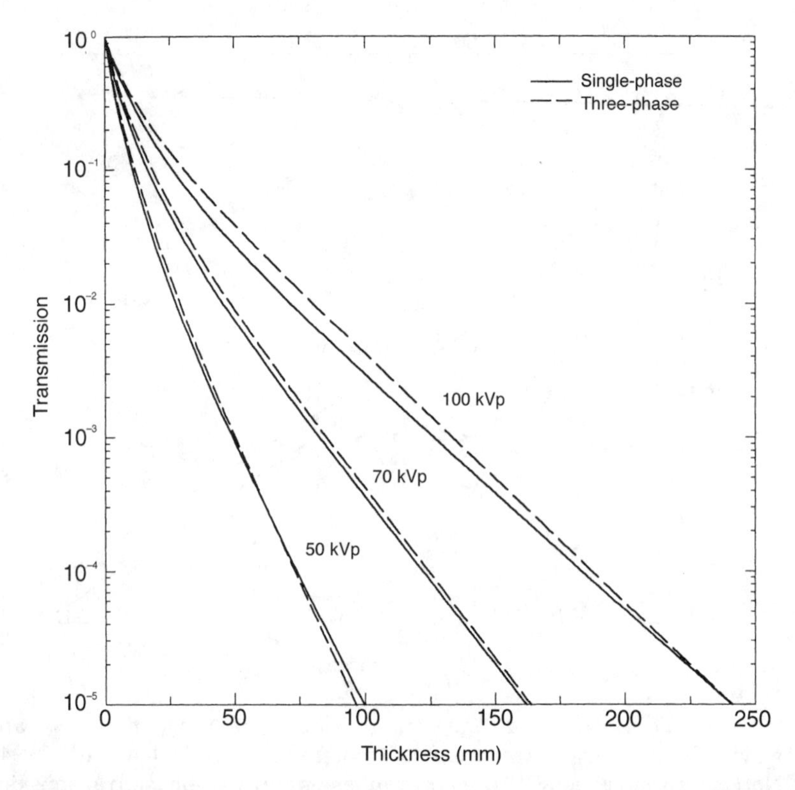

Fig. F.8. Barrier transmission for plate glass as a function of kVp and waveform (data are plotted from parameters given by Archer *et al.*, 1994). Note that the crossing of the single-phase and three-phase transmission curves for 50 kVp is the result of curve fitting for data that extended only to a transmission of 10^{-3}. The three-phase transmission curves also apply to constant-potential waveforms.

F.3.1 *Primary Radiation*

The primary beam is the intense, collimated radiation field that emanates from the x-ray port and is incident upon the patient and image receptor. Figure F.2 illustrates a primary protective barrier B in the useful beam that attenuates the beam before it reaches a person located at C. In most situations, the primary beam also is attenuated by the patient before impinging on the primary barrier. The theory of shielding primary radiation from diagnostic x-ray facilities has been discussed by Dixon and Simpkin (1998) and by the NCRP (in press).

Let $K_W(V_t)$ be the air kerma per unit workload in the primary beam at 1 m from the x-ray source operated at potential V_t. Values

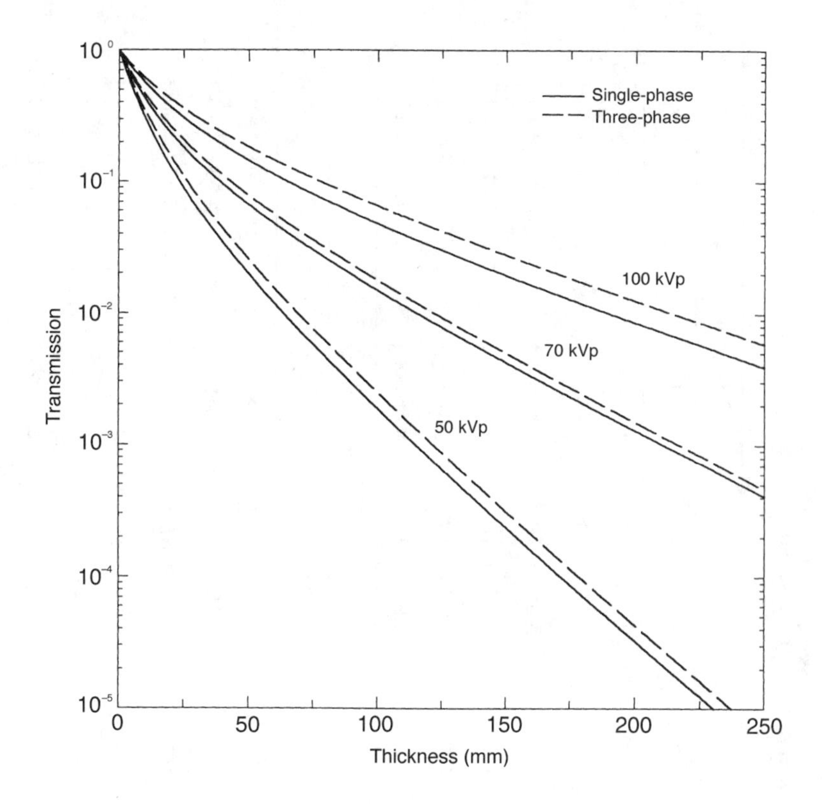

Fig. F.9. Barrier transmission for gypsum wallboard as a function of kVp and waveform (data are plotted from parameters given by Archer *et al.*, 1994). The three-phase transmission curves also apply to constant-potential waveforms.

of $K_W(V_t)$ for individual x-ray tubes will depend on generator waveform, anode material, filtration and anode angle. It can be shown (NCRP, in press) that for three-phase 12-pulse tungsten anode machines, the air kerma per workload (in units of mGy mA^{-1} min^{-1}) follows a cubic equation in operating potential V_t (*i.e.*, the kVp):

$$K_W(V_t) = 1.222 - (5.664 \times 10^{-2})\, V_t + (1.227 \times 10^{-3})\, V_t^{\,2} - (3.136 \times 10^{-6})\, V_t^{\,3}. \qquad \text{(F.8)}$$

For single-phase full-wave rectified tungsten machines, the air kerma per workload (in units of mGy mA^{-1} min^{-1}) is lower but also follows a cubic equation:

TABLE F.4a—*Barrier transmission parameters for three-phase or constant-potential waveforms.*[a]

kVp	Lead			Concrete		
	α (mm^{-1})	β (mm^{-1})	γ	α (mm^{-1})	β (mm^{-1})	γ
50	8.801	2.728×10^{1}	2.957×10^{-1}	9.032×10^{-2}	1.712×10^{-1}	2.324×10^{-1}
60	6.951	2.489×10^{1}	4.198×10^{-1}	6.251×10^{-2}	1.692×10^{-1}	2.733×10^{-1}
70	5.369	2.349×10^{1}	5.881×10^{-1}	5.087×10^{-2}	1.696×10^{-1}	3.847×10^{-1}
80	4.040	2.169×10^{1}	7.187×10^{-1}	4.583×10^{-2}	1.549×10^{-1}	4.926×10^{-1}
90	3.067	1.883×10^{1}	7.726×10^{-1}	4.228×10^{-2}	1.137×10^{-1}	4.690×10^{-1}
100	2.500	1.528×10^{1}	7.557×10^{-1}	3.925×10^{-2}	8.567×10^{-2}	4.273×10^{-1}
kVp	Gypsum Wallboard			Steel		
	α (mm^{-1})	β (mm^{-1})	γ	α (mm^{-1})	β (mm^{-1})	γ
50	3.883×10^{-2}	8.730×10^{-2}	5.105×10^{-1}	1.817	4.840	4.021×10^{-1}
60	2.985×10^{-2}	7.961×10^{-2}	6.169×10^{-1}	1.183	4.219	4.571×10^{-1}
70	2.302×10^{-2}	7.163×10^{-2}	7.299×10^{-1}	7.149×10^{-1}	3.798	5.378×10^{-1}
80	1.886×10^{-2}	6.093×10^{-2}	8.103×10^{-1}	4.921×10^{-1}	3.428	6.427×10^{-1}
90	1.633×10^{-2}	5.039×10^{-2}	8.585×10^{-1}	3.971×10^{-1}	2.913	7.204×10^{-1}
100	1.466×10^{-2}	4.171×10^{-2}	8.939×10^{-1}	3.415×10^{-1}	2.420	7.645×10^{-1}

kVp	Plate Glass			Wood		
	α (mm^{-1})	β (mm^{-1})	γ	α (mm^{-1})	β (mm^{-1})	γ
50	9.721×10^{-2}	1.799×10^{-1}	4.912×10^{-1}	1.076×10^{-2}	1.862×10^{-3}	1.170
60	7.452×10^{-2}	1.539×10^{-1}	5.304×10^{-1}	9.512×10^{-3}	9.672×10^{-4}	1.333
70	5.791×10^{-2}	1.357×10^{-1}	5.967×10^{-1}	8.550×10^{-3}	5.390×10^{-4}	1.194
80	4.955×10^{-2}	1.208×10^{-1}	7.097×10^{-1}	7.903×10^{-3}	8.640×10^{-4}	9.703×10^{-1}
90	4.550×10^{-2}	1.077×10^{-1}	8.522×10^{-1}	7.511×10^{-3}	1.159×10^{-3}	1.081
100	4.278×10^{-2}	9.466×10^{-2}	9.791×10^{-1}	7.230×10^{-3}	9.343×10^{-4}	1.309

[a]Condensed from Simpkin (1995).

TABLE F.4b—*Barrier transmission parameters for single-phase waveforms*[a]

kVp	Lead			Steel		
	α (mm^{-1})	β (mm^{-1})	γ	α (mm^{-1})	β (mm^{-1})	γ
50	6.046	3.290×10^{1}	2.537×10^{-1}	1.642	6.073	4.118×10^{-1}
70	4.241	2.683×10^{1}	4.814×10^{-1}	7.744×10^{-1}	5.243	6.268×10^{-1}
100	2.029	1.315×10^{-2}	4.835×10^{-1}	3.695×10^{-1}	3.663	8.572×10^{-1}
kVp	Plate Glass			Gypsum Wallboard		
	α (mm^{-1})	β (mm^{-1})	γ	α (mm^{-1})	β (mm^{-1})	γ
50	8.721×10^{-2}	2.221×10^{-1}	4.430×10^{-1}	3.856×10^{-2}	1.078×10^{-1}	5.047×10^{-1}
70	5.713×10^{-2}	1.693×10^{-1}	6.117×10^{-1}	2.245×10^{-2}	8.524×10^{-1}	7.112×10^{-1}
100	3.984×10^{-2}	1.058×10^{-1}	6.793×10^{-1}	1.478×10^{-2}	5.277×10^{-1}	8.006×10^{-1}
kVp	Lead acrylic			Wood		
	α (mm^{-1})	β (mm^{-1})	γ	α (mm^{-1})	β (mm^{-1})	γ
50	3.657	1.962×10^{1}	3.260×10^{-1}	1.131×10^{-2}	3.770×10^{-3}	1.133
70	2.588	1.380×10^{1}	5.063×10^{-1}	9.010×10^{-3}	1.610×10^{-3}	1.176
100	2.796	1.138×10^{1}	6.342×10^{-1}	7.200×10^{-3}	9.500×10^{-4}	1.207

[a]Condensed from Archer *et al.* (1994). Note that Archer *et al.* did not measure attenuation properties of concrete.

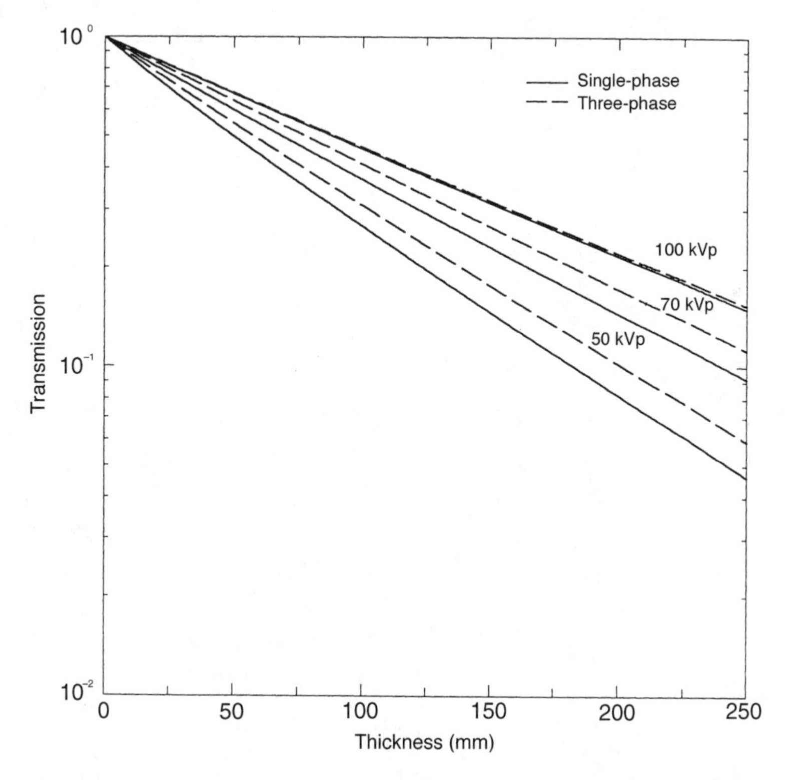

Fig. F.10. Barrier transmission for wood as a function of kVp and waveform (data are plotted from parameters given by Archer *et al.*, 1994). The three-phase transmission curves also apply to constant-potential waveforms.

$$K_W(V_t) = -0.37 - (2.58 \times 10^{-3})\, V_t + (5.37 \times 10^{-4})\, V_t^2 - (1.02 \times 10^{-6})\, V_t^3 \,. \qquad \text{(F.9)}$$

Note that Equations F.8 and F.9 were derived from data taken from equipment typical of diagnostic radiology and are valid only in the range 50 to 150 kVp. The applicability of Equations F.8 and F.9 to dental x-ray equipment has been investigated by McDavid *et al.* (1999),[7] who reported good agreement with Equation F.9 for single-phase units. However, high frequency units were less well described by Equation F.8. Differences may be expected due to differences in beam quality arising from dissimilar added filtration.

[7]McDavid, D. (1999). Personal communication (University of Texas Health Science Center, San Antonio, Texas).

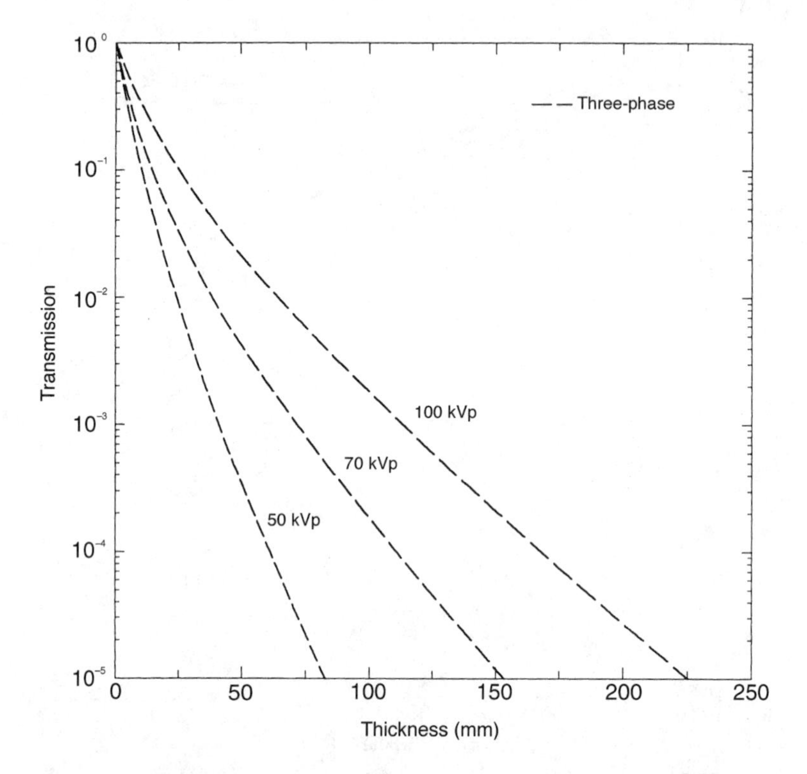

Fig. F.11. Barrier transmission for concrete as a function of kVp. Note that only three-phase data are available (data are plotted from parameters given in Simpkin, 1995). The three-phase transmission curves also apply to constant-potential waveforms.

For an occupied area shielded by a barrier of material m and thickness x having primary barrier transmission $B_{\mathrm{P}}(x,\mathrm{m},V_{\mathrm{t}})$, the air kerma to an occupied area at distance d_{P} away from a tube having workload $W(V_{\mathrm{t}})$ distributed so that just a fraction of the use factor (U) of its workload is directed toward a specified barrier, the total shielded primary air kerma K_{P} is:

$$K_{\mathrm{P}} = \frac{K_W(V_{\mathrm{t}})\ W(V_{\mathrm{t}})\ U}{d_{\mathrm{P}}^2}\ B_{\mathrm{P}}(x,\mathrm{m},V_{\mathrm{t}})\ . \qquad \text{(F.10)}$$

NCRP (in press) will include a discussion of the effect of attenuation by the image receptor and structures supporting the image receptor through the inclusion of an image receptor barrier thickness that is added to the wall barrier thickness. As a conservatively safe assumption, NCRP (in press) will not include patient attenuation for diagnostic radiology shielding calculations, since the patient occasionally does not intercept the primary beam. For intraoral dental radiography, the effect of patient attenuation may be included, since appropriate use of modern collimators ensures that the patient always intercepts the entire primary beam. NCRP Report No. 35 (NCRP, 1970) included the effect of shielding by the patient and image receptor by adjusting the use factor. For this Report, the effect of patient and image receptor attenuation for intraoral radiography is considered specifically by the multiplicative factor $a_{pt}(V_t)$, which is the average transmission through the patient with the image receptor in place for operating potential V_t. Examples of measured patient transmission factors are given in Figure F.4. Note that panoramic dental radiography units completely intercept the primary beam, such that no primary barrier calculations are required. Including the effect of patient and image receptor transmission, Equation F.10 then becomes:

$$K_P = \frac{K_W(V_t)\ W(V_t)\ a_{pt}(V_t)\ U}{d_P^2}\ B_P(x,\mathrm{m},V_t)\ . \qquad \text{(F.11)}$$

Calculations are simplest when the workload consists of a single, most prevalent, operating potential. If a unit is operated such that the workload is divided between several operating potentials (for instance half of the studies are done at 60 kVp and half at 90 kVp), a more accurate barrier calculation can be performed by considering each portion of the workload separately. The formalism for this detailed approach will be presented by NCRP (in press). For conservatively safe calculations (*i.e.*, resulting in greater shielding than may otherwise be necessary), one may assume that all the workload occurs at the highest clinically used operating potential. Note that the highest clinically used operating potential may be less than the highest operating potential that the unit can supply.

F.3.2 *Secondary Radiation*

Secondary radiation is an unavoidable consequence of the primary beam. Barriers that are never struck by the primary beam need to serve as adequate shields against scattered and leakage radiation. In some dental imaging situations, regulations and equipment design considerations result in the complete interception of the primary beam by an absorbing barrier behind or incorporated into the image receptor. This is the case for panoramic equipment. The air kerma in an occupied area from primary radiation is thus assumed nil, and that from scattered and leakage radiation will predominate. Figure F.3 illustrates a secondary protective barrier.

Here the barrier B attenuates the radiation leaking through the tube housing and that scattered from objects, such as the patient, in the path of the useful beam. The theory of shielding secondary radiation from diagnostic x-ray facilities has been discussed in Simpkin and Dixon (1998) and in NCRP (in press).

F.3.2.1 *Scattered Radiation.* The intensity of the x-radiation scattered off the patient through angle θ is dependent on θ, the number of primary photons incident on the patient, the primary photon energy, and the location of the x-ray beam on the patient. It is presumed that, all else being equal, the number of primary photons incident on the patient varies linearly with the x-ray beam area. Thus for fixed kVp, milliampere-seconds, and collimation, the scattered radiation intensity is independent of the distance from the source to the patient.

It can be shown (NCRP, in press) that the total weekly air kerma [$K_S(x,\mathrm{m},\theta)$] in a shielded area due to scattered radiation from a single source at operating potential V_t, is given by:

$$K_S(x,\mathrm{m},\theta) = \frac{a_1(\theta, V_t) \times 10^{-6}\ K_W(V_t)\,(1-U)\ W(V_t)}{d_S^2}\ B_P(x,\mathrm{m},V_t)\ \frac{F}{d_F^2}\,, \quad \text{(F.12)}$$

where $a_1(\theta,V_t)$ is the scaled scatter fraction per unit beam area (in units of cm^{-2}) at 1 m from the scattered radiation source, d_S is the distance (in meters) from the patient to the point of calculation, F is the primary field size (in units of cm^2) at d_F meters from the primary source, and other symbols are as previously described. The scaled scatter fraction for tungsten anode beams can be shown to be adequately described (NCRP, in press) by:

$$a_1(\theta,V_t) = (1.60 \times 10^{-2})\,(V_t - 125) + 8.434 - (1.105 \times 10^{-1})\,\theta + (9.828 \times 10^{-4})\,\theta^2 - (1.741 \times 10^{-6})\,\theta^3. \quad \text{(F.13)}$$

F.3.2.2 *Leakage Radiation.* The leakage air-kerma rate [$\dot{K}_L(V_t)$] from the x-ray tube operating at potential V_t and time t, is proportional to V_t^2, the x-ray current occurring at this potential at this moment [$I(V_t,t)$] and a transmission factor $B_{Pb}(x_H,V_t)$ for x-ray penetration through the tube housing of lead thickness x_H. Then, 1 m from the source:

$$\dot{K}_L(V_t) = \mathrm{C}\ V_t^2\ B_{Pb}(x_H,V_t)\ I(V_t,t), \quad \text{(F.14)}$$

where C is a constant.

As discussed above, current regulations in the United States require that the exposure rate due to leakage radiation not exceed 0.1 R h^{-1} at a distance of 1 m from the source (equivalent to an air-kerma rate of 0.876 mGy h^{-1}), when the tube is operated at its maximum leakage technique factors of $V_{t,max}$ and I_{max}. International regulations (IEC, 1994) require that leakage radiation from dental intraoral x-ray tube assemblies not exceed 0.25 mGy in 1 h at a distance of 1 m from the source, when the tube is operated at its maximum duty cycle. The thickness of lead required for various leakage technique factors has been reviewed (Simpkin and Dixon, 1998). For instance, for a tungsten anode tube operated at 100 kVp and 5 mA, about 2 mm of lead is required in the x-ray housing. When operated at other technique factors, particularly at lower kVp, considerably less than the maximum leakage radiation is produced. For example, for an x-ray tube housing with leakage technique factors 100 kVp and 5 mA and shielded by 2 mm of lead, the leakage radiation at a clinical operating potential of 70 kVp is about 0.3 percent of the maximum leakage.

NCRP (in press) has shown that the leakage air kerma from a housing designed to the U.S. standard (100 mR h^{-1} at 1 m) (*i.e.*, an air-kerma rate of 1.46×10^{-2} mGy min^{-1}) at a point shielded by a barrier of thickness x and material m, for a tube operated at potential V_t, is given by:

$$K_L(x,\mathrm{m}) = (1.46 \times 10^{-2}) \frac{V_t^2 \; B_{Pb}(x_H, V_t)}{V_{t,max}^2 \; B_{Pb}(x_H, V_{t,max}) \; I_{max} \; d_L^2} \; e^{\left[\frac{-0.693x}{x_{1/2}(\mathrm{m}, V_{t,max})}\right]} (1 - U) \; W(V_t) \; . \qquad \text{(F.15)}$$

For housings designed to the international standard, the constant 1.46×10^{-2} mGy min^{-1} is replaced by 4.17×10^{-3} mGy min^{-1} (0.25 mGy per 60 min). For tubes not rated for continuous operation, the value of I_{max} is the average current in 1 h when the tube is operated at its maximum duty cycle.

F.4 Examples of Barrier Calculations

F.4.1 *Example of a Primary Barrier Exact Calculation*

The required barrier thickness of a lateral wall is calculated during the architectural design of an intraoral dental radiography suite. The room contains a high frequency dental radiography unit to be used exclusively for intraoral studies. All patients will be imaged using E-speed film and a 40 cm cone. To be conservatively safe, all procedures are assumed to be performed at 90 kVp. The workload is not known, so a "high volume" is assumed to ensure the room would not be under-shielded. Using Table F.3, a workload of 13 mA min week^{-1} is used. The wall to be shielded is lateral to the patient and is assumed to have a use factor (U) of 0.4 (from Table F.2). A patient transmission factor [$a_{pt}(V_t)$] of 0.1 (from Figure F.4) is assumed. The primary barrier wall 2 m distant from the tube head separates the intraoral radiography room from an office (T = 1) occupied by a secretary or receptionist and members of the public.

Since only primary radiation is to be considered, Equation F.2 may be set equal to Equation F.11 and solved for B_P (x,m,V_t) as:

$$B_P(x,\mathrm{m},V_t) = \frac{P\,d_P^2}{K_W(V_t)\;W(V_t)\;a_{pt}(V_t)\;U\,T} , \qquad \text{(F.16)}$$

where $K_W(V_t)$ for high frequency equipment is approximated by Equation F.8 with V_t = 90 kVp, and P is 0.02 mGy week^{-1}. Inserting these values, $K_W(90)$ = 3.775 mGy mA^{-1} min^{-1} and $B_P(x,\mathrm{m},90)$, the required barrier transmission is calculated to be 4.07×10^{-2}. Equation F.5 may then be used to solve for the required thickness of material resulting in the requisite barrier transmission. Using Table F.4a at 90 kVp, the barrier transmission coefficients are as follows: for lead, $\alpha(90) = 3.067$, $\beta(90) = 1.883 \times 10^{1}$, and $\gamma(90) = 7.726 \times 10^{-1}$; for gypsum wallboard, $\alpha(90) = 1.633 \times 10^{-2}$, $\beta(90) = 5.039 \times 10^{-2}$, and $\gamma(90) = 8.585 \times 10^{-1}$. Substituting these coefficients and the previously obtained value for $B_P(x,\mathrm{m},90)$ into Equation F.5, the required thickness is calculated to be 0.39 mm of lead or 109 mm of gypsum wallboard. Note that this calculation ignores the leakage and scattered radiations due to the fraction of the workload that the tube is not oriented toward this primary barrier. Including the effects of leakage and scattered radiation increases the air-kerma incident on the barrier by about 10 percent. To maintain the shielding design goal of 0.02 mGy week^{-1}, the thickness of lead needs to be increased to 0.41 mm and the thickness of gypsum wallboard increased to 115 mm.

F.4.2 *Example of an Open Space Design Calculation*

During the design phase of a dental suite, it is proposed to place two procedure chairs in the same room, such that they can share the same intraoral equipment. The chairs are to be parallel and

2 m apart, separated by an opaque, but otherwise radiolucent barrier. The high frequency equipment operates at 70 or 100 kVp and 10 mA. To provide a conservatively safe calculation, it is assumed that all procedures are performed at 100 kVp and a "heavy" workload of 12 mA min week^{-1}. The primary, scattered and leakage air kermas are calculated with Equations F.2, F.11, F.12 and F.15 under the following assumptions: the barrier thickness is zero, the use factor is 0.4 (since the chairs are parallel), the occupancy factor is one, the patient transmission factor is 0.1, and the tube is always operated at its maximum leakage technique factors of 100 kVp and average leakage current in 1 h of 0.5 mA. Under these conditions the air kermas due to primary, scattered and leakage radiations are 0.563, 0.012 and 0.053 mGy week^{-1}, for a total of 0.63 mGy week^{-1}. However, the same patient will not be present for all procedures in an entire week. A more reasonable assumption is that a given patient might be present for 1/20 to 1/10 of the workload, for a total air-kerma range of 0.03 to 0.06 mGy week^{-1}, which exceeds the shielding design goal of 0.02 mGy week^{-1} for uncontrolled areas. To reduce the air-kerma level from one procedure area to the other to the shielding design goal, the radiolucent barrier needs to be modified so that it contains at least 0.08 mm of lead, 2.6 cm of gypsum wallboard, or 1.1 cm of plate glass.

This design would also exceed the shielding design goal for a controlled area (0.1 mGy week^{-1}) for a worker who might be present in the room a significant portion of the time (and positioned in the path of the primary beam), since the total air kerma is 0.63 mGy week^{-1}. Any physical layout that permits simultaneous accommodation of two patients in one room may also permit unnecessary or excessive occupational exposure. For example, a member of the occupationally-exposed staff may expose a radiograph for one patient while a second member of the staff is attending the second patient in the room. It is usual radiology practice that no one but the patient should be in the room at the time of exposure of static image receptors such as for dental radiographs. An appropriate barrier between the two chairs is the most effective remedy for both the second patient and the dental worker.

Alternatively, since many intraoral imaging views are lateral or oblique, simply orienting the chairs back to back will greatly reduce the amount of primary radiation that one chair receives from the other. If a use factor of 0.2 is assumed for the anterioposterior or posteroanterior orientation, the primary air kerma would be cut in half, and a new evaluation could be made to see if the P values for controlled and uncontrolled areas are met. The use of the vertical beam technique with the patient reclined would further reduce the use factor to near zero for periapical but not bitewing radiography (Section 3.1.4.1.3).

F.5 Examples of Approximate Barrier Thickness Calculations

In some situations accurate calculations may not be possible (due for instance to unavailability of all necessary information) or a conservatively safe (thicker) barrier calculation may be desired. In this case, the simplified techniques discussed below may be used. The basis for this method is to make simplifying assumptions and to convert the results of application of the exact technique to table form.

Tables F.5 to F.10 are the results of exact calculations of required barrier thickness for primary and secondary (leakage plus scattered) radiation. The following assumptions have been made in generating Tables F.5 to F.10. For leakage radiation, the instantaneous tube current is assumed to be 10 mA regardless of kVp and the duty cycle is assumed to be 1/20, resulting in an effective leakage current of 0.5 mA. Housing leakage is assumed to just meet the leakage radiation standard at the kVp given in the lookup column. (This assumption will always result in an overestimate of leakage radiation for housings designed to meet the standard at a higher kVp than they are typically operated.) The scattered radiation area is assumed to be 46 cm^2 and the distance to the scattered radiation volume is assumed to be 40 cm (long cone). The scattering angle is assumed to be 90 degrees. The workload is assumed to be incurred at the same kVp.

F.5.1 *Shielding Tables for Various Barrier Materials*

Tables F.5 to F.10, list the thickness required for primary and secondary protective barriers of lead, gypsum wallboard, and solid concrete that were calculated on the basis of the assumptions given above. Table F.11 lists the properties of several common building materials. Studies have been made of several commonly used wall sections to determine their transmission properties for primary and secondary dental x rays (MacDonald *et al.*, 1983). Systematic studies of the properties of a wide range of materials used for shielding diagnostic x rays have been reported (Archer *et al.*, 1994; Simpkin, 1995). The results of these studies are summarized in

Tables F.4a and F.4b. Shielding properties depend upon the waveform of the incident x rays, with greater thickness required for constant-potential equipment. Note that, compared to earlier (now obsolete) reports such as NCRP Reports No. 35 and No. 49 (NCRP, 1970; 1976), the data given in this Report are more representative of the beam quality (particularly added filtration standards) now in use.

F.5.2 *Use of Simplified Barrier Thickness Tables*

Shielding requirements of a dental office can be derived from a determination of the following parameters:

1. the maximum kVp at which the machine is operated
2. the distance from the source of radiation (x-ray tube) to position of interest
3. the weekly workload (milliampere-minutes per week)
4. the occupancy factor (Table F.1)
5. the leakage radiation characteristics of the unit

The following examples illustrate the use of barrier thickness tables.

F.5.2.1 *Example I.* A member of the public frequently spends half of his workday in a room directly below a dental x-ray room. When standing, the upper part of his body can come within 2 m of the x-ray source. The x-ray machine uses a constant-potential waveform, is operated only at 70 kVp, and is designed to meet the 0.25 mGy h^{-1} leakage radiation standard. The maximum weekly workload is estimated to be 32 mA min. The minimum floor thickness is 5 cm of concrete [density 2.4 g cm^{-3} (147 lb ft^{-3})]. Is the shielding adequate?

Conditions:

Type of barrier:	Secondary
Occupancy factor:	1/2
Shielding design goal:	Uncontrolled area, P = 0.02 mGy $week^{-1}$
Minimum distance from source:	2 m
Operating potential:	70 kVp (constant potential)
Workload:	32 mA min $week^{-1}$
Barrier material and thickness	Concrete, 5.1 cm (2 in)

TABLE F.5—*Primary barrier thickness for single-phase units.*[a]

$a_{pt}WUT$ (mA min week^{-1})	Distance (m)																				
8		1.00			1.41			2.00			2.83			4.00			5.66			8.00	
4					1.00			1.41			2.00			2.83			4.00			5.66	
2								1.00			1.41			2.00			2.83			4.00	
1											1.00			1.41			2.00			2.83	
0.5														1.00			1.41			2.00	
0.25																	1.00			1.41	
0.125																				1.00	
kVp	50	70	90	50	70	90	50	70	90	50	70	90	50	70	90	50	70	90	50	70	90
Controlled areas (P = 0.1)																					
Lead (mm)	0.16	0.40	1.10	0.12	0.31	0.87	0.09	0.23	0.67	0.06	0.16	0.49	0.04	0.10	0.35	0.02	0.06	0.23	0.00	0.03	0.14
Concrete (cm)	2.05	4.19	8.58	1.62	3.33	7.14	1.23	2.56	5.79	0.86	1.88	4.53	0.53	1.28	3.39	0.23	0.78	2.37	0.00	0.36	1.49
Gypsum wallboard (cm)	5.21	12.57	25.87	3.95	9.89	21.40	2.84	7.42	17.09	1.88	5.23	13.01	1.08	3.38	9.31	0.43	1.91	6.10	0.00	0.80	3.50
Steel (mm)	0.96	2.63	8.01	0.72	1.99	6.32	0.52	1.44	4.74	0.35	0.98	3.35	0.20	0.62	2.19	0.08	0.34	1.30	0.00	0.14	0.68
Plate glass (cm)	2.27	4.98	9.63	1.74	3.96	8.00	1.26	3.02	6.45	0.85	2.17	4.98	0.50	1.44	3.64	0.20	0.84	2.45	0.00	0.37	1.46

Uncontrolled areas (P = 0.02)

Lead (mm)	0.26	0.67	1.71	0.21	0.55	1.43	0.17	0.44	1.17	0.13	0.34	0.94	0.10	0.25	0.73	0.07	0.18	0.55	0.04	0.12	0.39
Concrete (cm)	3.15	6.48	12.18	2.65	5.45	10.59	2.19	4.48	9.06	1.75	3.60	7.60	1.35	2.80	6.21	0.98	2.09	4.92	0.63	1.47	3.75
Gypsum wallboard (cm)	8.55	19.26	36.54	7.05	16.32	31.91	5.64	13.46	27.33	4.34	10.73	22.83	3.18	8.19	18.46	2.18	5.90	14.29	1.32	3.94	10.45
Steel (mm)	1.61	4.37	12.20	1.31	3.59	10.37	1.04	2.86	8.58	0.79	2.19	6.85	0.58	1.61	5.23	0.40	1.12	3.77	0.24	0.72	2.53
Plate glass (cm)	3.68	7.55	13.53	3.05	6.42	11.83	2.45	5.32	10.16	1.90	4.28	8.52	1.41	3.31	6.94	0.98	2.43	5.44	0.60	1.66	4.05

[a]The shielding design goal (P) is given in units of milligray (air kerma) per week. Since single-phase concrete attenuation data were not available, constant-potential attenuation parameters were used for the generation of the concrete section of this table.

TABLE F.6—*Primary barrier thickness for constant-potential units.*[a]

$a_{pt}WUT$ (mA min week^{-1})										Distance (m)											
8		1.00			1.41			2.00			2.83			4.00			5.66			8.00	
4					1.00			1.41			2.00			2.83			4.00			5.66	
2								1.00			1.41			2.00			2.83			4.00	
1											1.00			1.41			2.00			2.83	
0.5														1.00			1.41			2.00	
0.25																	1.00			1.41	
0.125																				1.00	
kVp	50	70	90	50	70	90	50	70	90	50	70	90	50	70	90	50	70	90	50	70	90
Controlled areas (P = 0.1)																					
Lead (mm)	0.20	0.49	1.37	0.16	0.39	1.12	0.12	0.29	0.88	0.09	0.21	0.66	0.06	0.14	0.46	0.03	0.09	0.30	0.01	0.04	0.18
Concrete (cm)	2.32	4.57	9.17	1.87	3.68	7.70	1.46	2.87	6.31	1.08	2.15	5.01	0.73	1.52	3.82	0.41	0.98	2.76	0.11	0.53	1.82
Gypsum wallboard (cm)	6.57	14.41	30.31	5.18	11.66	25.67	3.90	9.05	21.11	2.75	6.65	16.68	1.76	4.54	12.48	0.93	2.77	8.64	0.25	1.38	5.33
Steel (mm)	1.18	3.17	9.65	0.92	2.48	7.81	0.70	1.86	6.07	0.50	1.34	4.49	0.32	0.90	3.13	0.17	0.55	2.02	0.05	0.28	1.17
Plate glass (cm)	2.78	5.71	11.10	2.21	4.66	9.50	1.68	3.66	7.91	1.20	2.74	6.34	0.78	1.92	4.83	0.41	1.22	3.41	0.11	0.63	2.15

Uncontrolled areas (P = 0.02)

Lead (mm)	0.31	0.75	1.99	0.26	0.64	1.72	0.21	0.52	1.45	0.17	0.42	1.20	0.13	0.32	0.95	0.10	0.24	0.72	0.06	0.16	0.52
Concrete (cm)	3.46	6.94	12.81	2.95	5.88	11.21	2.47	4.88	9.66	2.01	3.96	8.16	1.59	3.12	6.74	1.20	2.37	5.42	0.84	1.72	4.19
Gypsum wallboard (cm)	10.16	21.12	41.21	8.57	18.19	36.50	7.05	15.32	31.81	5.61	12.53	27.16	4.29	9.87	22.57	3.11	7.40	18.09	2.06	5.19	13.80
Steel (mm)	1.85	5.01	14.17	1.54	4.18	12.20	1.26	3.41	10.26	1.00	2.69	8.39	0.77	2.05	6.61	0.56	1.50	4.98	0.37	1.03	3.54
Plate glass (cm)	4.23	8.31	14.85	3.59	7.17	13.23	2.97	6.06	11.62	2.39	4.99	10.01	1.85	3.97	8.42	1.35	3.03	6.84	0.91	2.17	5.31

[a]The shielding design goal (P) is given in units of milligray (air kerma) per week.

TABLE F.7—*Secondary barrier thickness for single-phase units with 0.876 mGy* h^{-1} *(0.1 R* h^{-1}*) leakage.*[a]

$W(1-U)T$ (mA min $week^{-1}$)	Distance (m)																				
128		1.00			1.41			2.00			2.83			4.00			5.66			8.00	
64					1.00			1.41			2.00			2.83			4.00			5.66	
32								1.00			1.41			2.00			2.83			4.00	
16											1.00			1.41			2.00			2.83	
8														1.00			1.41			2.00	
4																	1.00			1.41	
2																				1.00	
kVp	50	70	100	50	70	100	50	70	100	50	70	100	50	70	100	50	70	100	50	70	100
Controlled areas (*P* = 0.1)																					
Lead (mm)	0.60	0.85	1.78	0.48	0.69	1.44	0.37	0.53	1.10	0.25	0.36	0.76	0.14	0.20	0.42	0.03	0.04	0.10	0.00	0.00	0.00
Concrete (cm)	4.00	7.10	9.24	3.23	5.74	7.48	2.47	4.38	5.73	1.70	3.02	3.98	0.94	1.67	2.26	0.18	0.36	0.63	0.00	0.00	0.00
Gypsum wallboard (cm)	9.37	16.12	24.61	7.57	13.04	19.93	5.78	9.95	15.26	3.98	6.88	10.60	2.19	3.81	5.98	0.43	0.82	1.59	0.00	0.00	0.00
Steel (mm)	2.20	4.67	9.80	1.78	3.77	7.93	1.36	2.88	6.06	0.94	1.99	4.18	0.51	1.09	2.32	0.10	0.23	0.54	0.00	0.00	0.00
Plate glass (cm)	4.14	6.34	9.13	3.35	5.12	7.40	2.55	3.91	5.66	1.76	2.70	3.94	0.97	1.50	2.23	0.19	0.33	0.61	0.00	0.00	0.00

Uncontrolled areas (P = 0.02)																					
Lead (mm)	0.86	1.22	2.56	0.74	1.06	2.21	0.63	0.90	1.87	0.51	0.73	1.53	0.40	0.57	1.19	0.28	0.41	0.85	0.17	0.24	0.51
Concrete (cm)	5.74	10.19	13.24	4.97	8.83	11.47	4.20	7.47	9.71	3.44	6.11	7.95	2.67	4.74	6.19	1.90	3.38	4.44	1.14	2.03	2.71
Gypsum wallboard (cm)	13.44	23.12	35.23	11.65	20.03	30.55	9.85	16.94	25.86	8.05	13.86	21.18	6.26	10.77	16.50	4.46	7.69	11.83	2.67	4.62	7.20
Steel (mm)	3.16	6.70	14.05	2.74	5.80	12.18	2.31	4.91	10.30	1.89	4.01	8.43	1.47	3.12	6.55	1.05	2.22	4.68	0.63	1.33	2.82
Plate glass (cm)	5.94	9.08	13.07	5.15	7.87	11.33	4.36	6.66	9.59	3.56	5.45	7.86	2.77	4.23	6.13	1.97	3.03	4.40	1.18	1.82	2.68

[a]The shielding design goal (P) is given in units of milligray (air kerma) per week. The leakage technique factors assumed 0.5 mA aver age leakage current with sufficient housing shielding to just meet the leakage standard at the kVp indicated in the column. The scattered radiation area is assumed to be 46 cm^2 and the distance to the scattered radiation volume is assumed to be 40 cm (long cone).

TABLE F.8—*Secondary barrier thickness for constant-potential units with 0.876 mGy h^{-1} (0.1 R h^{-1}) leakage.*[a]

$W(1-U)T$ (mA min week^{-1})	Distance (m)																				
128		1.00			1.41			2.00			2.83			4.00			5.66			8.00	
64					1.00			1.41			2.00			2.83			4.00			5.66	
32								1.00			1.41			2.00			2.83			4.00	
16											1.00			1.41			2.00			2.83	
8														1.00			1.41			2.00	
4																	1.00			1.41	
2																				1.00	
kVp	50	70	100	50	70	100	50	70	100	50	70	100	50	70	100	50	70	90	50	70	100
Controlled areas (*P* = 0.1)																					
Lead (mm)	0.41	0.68	1.46	0.33	0.55	1.18	0.26	0.42	0.90	0.18	0.29	0.63	0.10	0.16	0.35	0.02	0.04	0.10	0.00	0.00	0.00
Concrete (cm)	4.01	7.12	9.28	3.24	5.76	7.52	2.48	4.40	5.77	1.71	3.05	4.03	0.95	1.70	2.32	0.20	0.40	0.71	0.00	0.00	0.00
Gypsum wallboard (cm)	9.34	15.79	25.03	7.55	12.78	20.31	5.77	9.77	15.60	3.99	6.78	10.91	2.22	3.80	6.28	0.47	0.91	1.88	0.00	0.00	0.00
Steel (mm)	1.99	5.07	10.65	1.61	4.10	8.62	1.23	3.13	6.59	0.85	2.17	4.57	0.47	1.20	2.57	0.10	0.27	0.68	0.00	0.00	0.00
Plate glass (cm)	3.73	6.28	8.62	3.02	5.08	7.00	2.31	3.89	5.39	1.60	2.70	3.78	0.89	1.51	2.19	0.19	0.37	0.67	0.00	0.00	0.00

Uncontrolled areas (P = 0.02)

Lead (mm)	0.59	0.98	2.10	0.52	0.85	1.82	0.44	0.72	1.54	0.36	0.59	1.27	0.28	0.46	0.99	0.20	0.33	0.71	0.12	0.20	0.44
Concrete (cm)	5.79	10.28	13.36	5.02	8.92	11.59	4.25	7.55	9.83	3.49	6.19	8.07	2.72	4.83	6.32	1.95	3.47	4.57	1.19	2.12	2.85
Gypsum wallboard (cm)	13.47	22.76	35.97	11.68	19.75	31.25	9.90	16.74	26.52	8.12	13.73	21.80	6.33	10.73	17.09	4.55	7.72	12.39	2.78	4.73	7.74
Steel (mm)	2.88	7.31	15.35	2.50	6.35	13.32	2.12	5.38	11.29	1.73	4.41	9.26	1.35	3.44	7.23	0.97	2.47	5.21	0.59	1.51	3.20
Plate glass (cm)	5.38	9.05	12.37	4.67	7.85	10.75	3.96	6.65	9.13	3.24	5.46	7.51	2.53	4.26	5.90	1.82	3.07	4.29	1.11	1.89	2.69

[a]The shielding design goal (P) is given in units of milligray (air kerma) per week. The leakage technique factors assumed 0.5 mA aver age leakage current with sufficient housing shielding to just meet the leakage standard at the kVp indicated in the column. The scattered radiation area is assumed to be 46 cm^2 and the distance to the scattered radiation volume is assumed to be 40 cm (long cone).

TABLE F.9—*Secondary barrier thickness for single-phase units with 0.25 mGy h^{-1} leakage.*[a]

$W(1-U)T$ (mA min $week^{-1}$)	Distance (m)																				
128		1.00			1.41			2.00			2.83			4.00			5.66			8.00	
64					1.00			1.41			2.00			2.83			4.00			5.66	
32								1.00			1.41			2.00			2.83			4.00	
16											1.00			1.41			2.00			2.83	
8														1.00			1.41			2.00	
4																	1.00			1.41	
2																				1.00	
kVp	50	70	100	50	70	100	50	70	100	50	70	100	50	70	100	50	70	100	50	70	100
Controlled areas (*P* = 0.1)																					
Lead (mm)	0.39	0.56	1.17	0.28	0.40	0.83	0.16	0.23	0.50	0.05	0.08	0.20	0.00	0.00	0.01	0.00	0.00	0.00	0.00	0.00	0.00
Concrete (cm)	2.62	4.66	6.19	1.86	3.31	4.48	1.10	1.98	2.82	0.37	0.72	1.30	0.00	0.00	0.07	0.00	0.00	0.00	0.00	0.00	0.00
Gypsum wallboard (cm)	6.14	10.65	16.62	4.36	7.59	12.01	2.58	4.56	7.49	0.84	1.66	3.28	0.00	0.00	0.15	0.00	0.00	0.00	0.00	0.00	0.00
Steel (mm)	1.44	3.06	6.49	1.02	2.17	4.63	0.60	1.29	2.80	0.19	0.44	1.07	0.00	0.00	0.03	0.00	0.00	0.00	0.00	0.00	0.00
Plate glass (cm)	2.72	4.19	6.18	1.93	2.99	4.48	1.14	1.80	2.82	0.38	0.67	1.27	0.00	0.00	0.07	0.00	0.00	0.00	0.00	0.00	0.00

Uncontrolled areas (P = 0.02)

lead (mm)	0.65	0.93	1.94	0.54	0.77	1.60	0.42	0.60	1.26	0.31	0.44	0.92	0.19	0.28	0.59	0.08	0.12	0.27	0.00	0.00	0.04
Concrete (cm)	4.35	7.74	10.14	3.59	6.38	8.39	2.82	5.02	6.65	2.06	3.67	4.93	1.30	2.33	3.25	0.56	1.04	1.68	0.00	0.00	0.36
Gypsum wallboard (cm)	10.21	17.63	27.19	8.41	14.54	22.51	6.62	11.47	17.86	4.83	8.40	13.23	3.05	5.36	8.68	1.29	2.40	4.34	0.00	0.00	0.80
Steel (mm)	2.40	5.09	10.73	1.97	4.19	8.86	1.55	3.30	6.99	1.13	2.41	5.13	0.71	1.52	3.28	0.30	0.66	1.50	0.00	0.00	0.19
Plate glass (cm)	4.51	6.93	10.09	3.72	5.72	8.36	2.93	4.51	6.63	2.14	3.30	4.93	1.35	2.11	3.25	0.57	0.96	1.66	0.00	0.00	0.33

[a]The shielding design goal (P) given in units of milligray (air kerma) per week. The leakage technique factors assumed 0.5 mA average leakage current with sufficient housing shielding to just meet the leakage standard at the kVp indicated in the column. The scattered radiation area is assumed to be 46 cm^2 and the distance to the scattered radiation volume is assumed to be 40 cm (long cone).

TABLE F.10—*Secondary barrier thickness for constant-potential units with 0.25 mGy h^{-1} leakage.*[a]

$W(1-U)T$ (mA min $week^{-1}$)	Distance (m)																				
128		1.00			1.41			2.00			2.83			4.00			5.66			8.00	
64					1.00			1.41			2.00			2.83			4.00			5.66	
32								1.00			1.41			2.00			2.83			4.00	
16											1.00			1.41			2.00			2.83	
8														1.00			1.41			2.00	
4																	1.00			1.41	
2																				1.00	
kVp	50	70	100	50	70	100	50	70	100	50	70	100	50	70	100	50	70	90	50	70	100
Controlled areas (*P* = 0.1)																					
Lead (mm)	0.27	0.45	0.98	0.19	0.32	0.70	0.11	0.19	0.43	0.04	0.07	0.19	0.00	0.00	0.02	0.00	0.00	0.00	0.00	0.00	0.00
Concrete (cm)	2.63	4.69	6.27	1.87	3.34	4.57	1.12	2.02	2.93	0.40	0.78	1.43	0.00	0.00	0.23	0.00	0.00	0.00	0.00	0.00	0.00
Gypsum wallboard (cm)	6.15	10.52	17.32	4.38	7.54	12.69	2.63	4.61	8.15	0.93	1.83	3.92	0.00	0.00	0.57	0.00	0.00	0.00	0.00	0.00	0.00
Steel (mm)	1.31	3.34	7.11	0.93	2.37	5.10	0.56	1.42	3.14	0.20	0.53	1.33	0.00	0.00	0.14	0.00	0.00	0.00	0.00	0.00	0.00
Plate glass (cm)	2.46	4.18	6.05	1.76	3.01	4.46	1.06	1.85	2.90	0.38	0.75	1.43	0.00	0.00	0.22	0.00	0.00	0.00	0.00	0.00	0.00

Uncontrolled areas (P = 0.02)

Lead (mm)	0.45	0.74	1.61	0.37	0.62	1.34	0.30	0.49	1.06	0.22	0.36	0.79	0.14	0.23	0.52	0.06	0.11	0.26	0.00	0.01	0.06
Concrete (cm)	4.40	7.83	10.29	3.64	6.47	8.55	2.88	5.12	6.81	2.11	3.77	5.10	1.36	2.43	3.44	0.63	1.16	1.88	0.00	0.11	0.57
Gypsum wallboard (cm)	10.28	17.47	28.20	8.49	14.46	23.49	6.72	11.46	18.80	4.94	8.48	14.14	3.18	5.53	9.57	1.46	2.67	5.20	0.00	0.24	1.47
Steel (mm)	2.19	5.58	11.79	1.81	4.61	9.76	1.43	3.64	7.74	1.05	2.68	5.73	0.67	1.72	3.75	0.31	0.80	1.87	0.00	0.06	0.41
Plate glass (cm)	4.11	6.94	9.79	3.40	5.75	8.17	2.69	4.56	6.56	1.98	3.38	4.96	1.28	2.21	3.39	0.59	1.08	1.88	0.00	0.11	0.56

[a]The shielding design goal (*P*) given in units of milligray (air kerma) per week. The leakage technique factors assumed 0.5 mA average leakage current with sufficient housing shielding to just meet the leakage standard at the kVp indicated in the column. The scattered radiation area is assumed to be 46 cm^2 and the distance to the scattered radiation volume is assumed to be 40 cm (long cone).

TABLE F.11—*Properties of common building materials.*

Material	Density (g cm^{-3})	Half-Value Layer (mm)[a]		
		50 kVp	70 kVp	100 kVp
Lead	11.35	0.08	0.13	0.28
Concrete	2.35	7.4	13.6	17.7
Gypsum wallboard	0.75	17.8	30.1	47.3
Steel	7.40	0.38	0.97	2.03
Plate glass	2.56	7.1	12.0	16.2
Wood	0.55	64.4	81.1	95.9

[a]Half-value layers ($x_{1/2}$) are for heavily filtered x-ray spectra from three-phase or constant-potential units. Half-value layers are calculated using the relationship $x_{1/2} = 0.693/\alpha$, where α is the fitting parameter for barrier transmission (Simpkin, 1995) from Table F.4a.

The solution may be found by referring to Table F.10 for secondary protective barriers. Since the tube is never directed at the floor ($U = 0$), all of the workload contributes to secondary radiation, and the product $W(1 - U)T$ is calculated to be 16 mA min week^{-1}. Locate this value in the left-most column. Read across to the right to the column indicating 2 m (in this case the second to the last column), then read down to the section labeled "Uncontrolled areas ($P = 0.02$)." Under the 70 kVp label within this distance column is the minimum barrier thickness of 1.16 cm of concrete. Since the existing barrier, 5.1 cm, exceeds 1.16, the existing barrier provides adequate protection for the conditions of occupancy in the room below the dental office. If the workload or other parameters change significantly, a new computation should be made.

F.5.2.2 *Example II.* Beyond one wall of this same dental office there is a corridor used by the general public. The wall is made of two slabs of 1.4 cm (5/8 inch) type "X" gypsum wallboard. The minimum distance to the x-ray source is 1 m. Does the wall provide adequate protection for persons using the corridor?

Conditions:

Type of barrier:	Primary
Occupancy factor:	1/5 (Table F.1)
Shielding design goal:	Uncontrolled area, $P = 0.02$ mGy week^{-1}
Minimum distance from source:	1 m
Operating potential:	70 kVp (constant potential)
Workload:	15 mA min week^{-1}
Barrier material and thickness	Gypsum wallboard, 2.8 cm

The minimum barrier thickness may be found by referring to Table F.6 for the primary protective barriers of constant-potential waveforms. In the absence of detailed use and patient transmission data, it is appropriate to assume that $a_{pt} = 0.1$ and $U = 0.4$. Thus the product $a_{pt}WUT$ is calculated to be 0.120 mA min week^{-1}. A value of 0.125 mA min week^{-1} may be used for table look up. Locate this value in the left-most column. Read across to the right to the column indicating 1 m (the last column), then read down to the section labeled "Uncontrolled areas ($P = 0.02$)". Under the 70 kVp label within the distance column is the minimum barrier thickness of 5.19 cm of gypsum wallboard. Secondary radiation also impinges on this barrier. Using Table F.10 with a $W(1 - U)T$ value of 1.8 mA min week^{-1} at 1 m and the same shielding design goal, the gypsum wallboard thickness for 2 mA min week^{-1} is 0.24 cm. Therefore, the 2.8 cm gypsum wallboard is enough for the secondary radiation, but not for the primary radiation. One way to provide adequate shielding for the primary radiation is to double the thickness of the gypsum wallboard.

F.5.2.3 *Example III*. In the design phase of a new intraoral imaging suite the barrier thickness of a wall between the imaging equipment and a waiting room is to be specified. The equipment is single phase, designed to meet the 0.25 mGy h^{-1} leakage standard and provides a maximum potential of 70 kVp. A workload of 32 mA min week^{-1} is assumed. The orientation of the equipment results in the wall being a primary barrier with a use factor of 0.4. Figure F.4 is used to estimate the patient transmission factor of 0.07. The waiting room lies directly on the other side of the wall, 1 m distant from the equipment.

Conditions:

Type of barrier:	Primary
Occupancy factor:	1 (Table F.1)
Shielding design goal:	Uncontrolled area, $P = 0.02$ mGy week^{-1}
Minimum distance from source:	1 m
Operating potential:	70 kVp (single phase)
Workload:	32 mA min week^{-1}

The minimum barrier thickness may be found by referring to Table F.5 for primary protective barriers of single-phase equipment. Since the product $a_{pt}WUT$ is calculated to be 0.9 mA min week^{-1}, a value of 1 mA min week^{-1} may be used for table lookup. Locate this value in the left-most column. Read across to the right to the column indicating 1 m (the fourth column from the left), then read down to the section labeled "Uncontrolled area ($P = 0.02$)". Under the 70 kVp label within the distance column is the minimum barrier thickness of 0.34 mm of lead or 10.73 cm of gypsum wallboard. Since the barrier thickness of gypsum wallboard would require eight slabs of type "X" gypsum wallboard (1.4 cm each), lead is the practical barrier material.

Secondary radiation also impinges upon this barrier. Table F.9 is used with a $W(1 - U)T$ value of 19 mA min week^{-1} at 1 m and the same shielding design goal ($P = 0.02$). However, at 1 m, Table F.9 has entries only for 16 and 32 mA min week^{-1}, with resulting shielding thicknesses of 0.44 and 0.60 mm of lead. Although not mathematically identical to the exact solution, a linear interpolation can be made between these two values to yield an approximate thickness of 0.47 mm of lead. The recommended thickness for secondary radiation should thus be somewhat greater than about 0.5 mm of lead. In fact, it is often difficult to obtain leaded wallboard with less than 0.79 mm (1/32 inch or 2 pounds per square foot) lead thickness. Hence the minimum practical lead thickness for this wall could be 0.79 mm, resulting in greater shielding than is required for either primary or secondary radiation.

F.6 Summary

As demonstrated in this Appendix, various techniques are available for calculations of required barrier thickness for dental installations. While varying degrees of sophistication may be used, the acceptability of upgraded existing or planned new barriers cannot be assumed. Particularly for new construction and typical circumstances, appropriate shielding adds little to the cost of construction. Also, there needs to be a performance assessment by a qualified expert to confirm that occupational and public effective dose limits will not be exceeded by the structural shielding design, prior to facility operation. The recommendations in this Report are applied to upgraded or new shielding designs, but not to existing barriers that otherwise met prior requirements.

Appendix G

Radiation Quantities and Units

NCRP presently expresses the values of radiation quantities in the International System of Units (le Systeme Internationale d'Unites, or SI units). These units have replaced the previously used units (Table G.1) in most of the scientific literature. The quantity exposure, previously expressed in roentgens (R), has been largely replaced by the quantity air kerma (K) (an acronym for kinetic energy released per unit mass), which is expressed in the same units as absorbed dose. However, some older instruments may provide readout only in roentgens; with others either SI or the previous units may be selected. Absorbed dose, the energy imparted by ionizing radiation to matter per unit mass, is expressed in gray (Gy) (the previous name was the rad). Equivalent dose, expressed in sievert (Sv) (the previous name was the rem), is used extensively in radiation protection. Equivalent dose is the mean absorbed dose in an organ or tissue modified by the radiation weighting factors for different types of radiation (*e.g.*, photons, neutrons, heavy charged particles). For diagnostic x rays (including dental), the radiation weighting factor is assigned the value of one, and absorbed dose in gray is numerically equal to equivalent dose in sievert

Another quantity, effective dose, is useful in comparing different dose distributions in the body. It takes into account the equivalent doses in radiosensitive organs or tissues, each modified by a tissue weighting factor that represents the relative contribution of risk of stochastic effect to that organ or tissue to total stochastic risk. The tissues receiving the higher doses in patients from dental radiography are portions of the active bone marrow, thyroid, bone surface of the skull, brain and salivary glands.

Conversion factors from the previous units to SI units are given in Table G.1. Detailed discussions of these concepts are given elsewhere (Bushberg *et al.*, 2001; ICRU, 1993; 1998; Johns and Cunningham, 1983; NCRP, 1985).

TABLE G.1—*Radiation quantities and units.*

Quantity	SI Units[a]		Previous Units[a]		Conversion
	Unit	Special Name	Unit	Special Name	
Exposure	C kg^{-1}	none	C kg^{-1}	roentgen (R)	1 R = 2.58×10^{-4} C kg^{-1}
Kerma; absorbed dose	J kg^{-1}	gray (Gy) 1 Gy = 1 J kg^{-1}	erg g^{-1}	rad 1 rad = 100 erg g^{-1}	1 Gy = 100 rad
Equivalent dose; effective dose	J kg^{-1}	sievert (Sv) 1 Sv = 1 J kg^{-1}	erg g^{-1}	rem 1 rem = 100 erg g^{-1}	1 Sv = 100 rem

[a]C = coulomb
J = joule
g = gram
kg = kilogram

Glossary

absorbed dose (*D*): The energy imparted by ionizing radiation to matter per unit mass of irradiated material at the point of interest. In the Systeme Internationale (SI), the unit is J kg^{-1}, given the special name gray (Gy). 1 Gy = 1 J kg^{-1}.

air kerma (*K*): (see **kerma**). Kerma in air. In this Report, the symbol K always refers to the quantity air kerma (in place of the usual symbol K_a), followed by an appropriate subscript to further describe the quantity (*e.g.*, K_P, air kerma from primary radiation).

ampere: Unit of electric current. One ampere is produced by 1 volt acting through a resistance of 1 ohm.

anode: The positive terminal of an x-ray tube. Typically, a tungsten block embedded in a copper stem and set at an angle to the cathode (the negative terminal of an x-ray tube, from which electrons are emitted). The anode emits x rays from the point of impact of the electron stream from the cathode.

area (or facility) dosimeter: A device used to estimate the absorbed dose or effective dose received by personnel, but not worn by an individual.

arthrography: Radiographic evaluation of a joint after injection of radiopaque contrast material into the joint space(s).

as low as reasonably achievable (ALARA): The principle of reducing the radiation dose of exposed persons to levels as low as is reasonably achievable, economic and social factors being taken into account.

attenuation: Loss of energy from a beam of ionizing radiation by scatter and absorption.

background: Ionizing radiation present in the region of interest and coming from sources other than that of primary concern (see also **natural background radiation**).

bisecting angle technique (bisect angle geometry): A technique for the radiographic exposure of intraoral image receptors whereby the central axis of the x-ray beam is directed at right angles to a plane determined by bisecting the angle formed by (1) the long axis of the tooth or teeth being imaged, and (2) the plane in which the image receptor is positioned behind the teeth.

bitewing radiograph: An intraoral radiograph that demonstrates the crowns, necks and coronal thirds of the roots of both upper and lower teeth. So named because the patient bites upon a tab or "wing" projecting from the center of the image-receptor packet.

cathode: (see **anode**).

cephalometer: A device used in obtaining cephalometric images. It consists of a source assembly, a connector arm, a head holder, and an image-receptor holder.

cephalometric radiography: Images of the head, primarily the dentofacial structures, usually obtained in lateral and posteroanterior orientation. Reproducible geometry is maintained by use of a cephalometer. The images are used to measure and study maxillofacial growth and maxilla-mandible relationships.

collimator (or beam-limiting device): A device that provides a means to restrict the dimensions of the useful beam.

computed tomography (CT): An imaging procedure that uses multiple x-ray transmission measurements and a computer program to generate tomographic images of the patient.

cone: (see **position indicating device**).

constant potential: The potential formed by a constant-voltage generator.

contrast:

subject contrast: the difference between two anatomic structures in attenuation of an x-ray beam or:

$$C = \frac{I_A - I_B}{I_B}, \qquad \text{(G.1)}$$

where C is subject contrast, and I_A and I_B are beam intensities after traversing structures A and B.

film contrast: the ability of a film (or other image receptor) to translate subject contrast to differences in the resulting image. Film contrast depends on both film characteristics and processing.

dental assistant: A member of the dental office staff whose principal duty is chair side assistance of the dentist in delivery of care. The assistant, properly trained, may be credentialed for exposure of dental radiographs.

dental hygienist: A member of the dental office staff whose principal duty is performing oral prophylaxis and related procedures; in the United States, a graduate of an accredited educational program in dental hygiene and registered in the state or political jurisdiction in which the practice is located. The dental hygiene curriculum includes training in radiography and the hygienist is credentialed to expose dental radiographs.

dental radiographic technologist: An individual who is trained and skilled in, and credentialed for, performing both routine and specialized radiographic examinations of the dentofacial region.

dentist: A graduate of an accredited dental institution with a degree of D.D.S., D.M.D. or equivalent.

deterministic effects: Effects that occur in all individuals who receive greater than the threshold dose and for which the severity of the effect varies with the dose.

detriment: The overall risk of radiation-induced health outcomes, including fatal and nonfatal cancer, genetic effects, and loss of life span from cancer and hereditary disease, weighted for severity and time of expression of the harmful effect, and averaged over both sexes and all ages in the population of interest (*i.e.*, general or working population).

diagnostic source assembly: A diagnostic source housing (x-ray tube housing) assembly with a beam-limiting device attached.

diagnostic reference level: A patient dose-related quantity per x-ray procedure or image that, if consistently exceeded in clinical practice, should elicit investigation and efforts for improved patient dose management.

digital radiography: A diagnostic procedure using an appropriate radiation source and imaging system that collects, processes, stores, recalls and presents image information in a digital array rather than on film.

dose: (see **absorbed dose**). Often used generically in place of a specific quantity, such as equivalent dose.

dose limit (annual): The maximum effective dose an individual may be permitted in any year from a given category of sources (*e.g.*, the occupational dose limit).

dosimetry: The science or technique of determining radiation dose.

dosimeter: Dose measuring device (see also **personal dosimeter** and **area dosimeter**).

effective dose (*E*): The sum of the weighted equivalent doses for the radiosensitive tissues and organs of the body. It is given by the expression:

$$E = \sum w_T H_T \ , \qquad \text{(G.2)}$$

where H_T is the equivalent dose in tissue or organ T and w_T is the tissue weighting factor for tissue T.

effective dose equivalent (H_E): An earlier formulation for effective dose (ICRP, 1977; NCRP, 1987b). Used in this Report only when values are quoted from the literature for this earlier quantity.

entrance air kerma (or entrance skin exposure): Air kerma (or exposure) measured free-in-air at the location of the entry surface of an irradiated person or phantom in the absence of the person or phantom.

equivalent dose (H_T): The mean absorbed dose in a tissue or organ modified by the radiation weighting factor (w_R) for the type and energy of radiation. The equivalent dose in tissue T is given by the expression:

$$H_T = \sum w_R (D_{T,R}) \ , \qquad \text{(G.3)}$$

where $D_{T,R}$ is the mean absorbed dose in the tissue or organ T due to radiation type R. The SI unit of equivalent dose is the J kg^{-1} with the special name sievert (Sv). 1 Sv = 1 J kg^{-1}.

exposure: A measure of the ionization produced in air by x or gamma radiation. The unit of exposure is coulomb per kilogram (C kg^{-1}) with the special name roentgen (R). Air kerma is often used in place of exposure. An exposure of 1 R corresponds to an air kerma of 8.76 mGy (see **kerma, gray, roentgen**).

field size: The geometrical projection of the x-ray beam on a plane perpendicular to the central ray of the distal end of the limiting diaphragm, as seen from the center of the front surface of the source.

film: A thin, transparent sheet of polyester or similar material coated on one or both sides with an emulsion sensitive to radiation and light.

direct exposure film: Film that is highly sensitive to the direct action of x rays rather than in combination with an intensifying screen.

screen film: Film whose light absorption characteristics are matched to the light emission characteristics of intensifying screens; screen film is not designed for use as direct exposure film.

film speed: For intraoral films, film speed is expressed as the reciprocal of the exposure (*i.e.*, R^{-1}) necessary to produce a density of one above base plus fog.

D-speed film: Direct exposure film with a speed range of 12 to 24 R^{-1}.

E-speed film: Direct exposure film with a speed range of 24 to 48 R^{-1}.

F-speed film: Direct exposure film with a speed range of 48 to 96 R^{-1}.

Faster films need less exposure (*i.e.*, a larger value of R^{-1}) to produce the same film density (*e.g.*, F-speed film is faster than E-speed film). For screen films, film speed is usually expressed in combination with an intensifying screen.

filter; filtration: Material in the useful beam that usually absorbs preferentially the less penetrating radiation. The total filtration consists of inherent and added filters.

inherent filtration: The filter permanently in the useful beam; it includes the window of the x-ray tube and any permanent enclosure for the tube or source.

added filtration: Filter in addition to the inherent filtration.

fluoroscopy: The process of producing a real-time image using x rays. The machine used for visualization, in which the dynamic image appears in real time on a display screen (usually video) is a fluoroscope. The fluoroscope can also produce a static record of an image formed on the output phosphor of an image intensifier. The image intensifier is an x-ray image receptor that increases the brightness of a fluoroscopic image by electronic amplification and image minification.

focal spot, effective: The apparent size of the radiation source region in a source assembly when viewed from the central axis of the useful radiation beam.

fog: A darkening of the whole or part of a radiograph by sources other than the radiation of the primary beam to which the film was exposed.

This can be due to chemicals in the processing solutions, light, or non-primary beam radiation.

geometric distortion: Distortion of the recorded image due to the combined optical effect of finite size of the focal spot and geometric separation of the anatomic area of interest from the image receptor and the focal spot.

genetic effects: Changes in reproductive cells that may result in detriment to offspring.

gray (Gy): The special name given to the SI unit of absorbed dose and kerma. 1 Gy = 1 J kg^{-1}.

grid: A device used to reduce scattered radiation reaching an image receptor during the making of a radiograph. It consists of a series of narrow (usually lead) strips closely spaced on their edges, separated by spacers of low density material.

half-value layer: Thickness of a specified substance that, when introduced into the path of a given beam of radiation, reduces the air-kerma rate (or exposure rate) by one-half.

hazardous chemical: Any chemical that is a physical hazard or a health hazard as defined by the Occupational Safety and Health Administration (OSHA, 1994a).

image receptor: A system for deriving a diagnostically usable image from the x rays transmitted through the patient. Examples: screen-film system, photostimulable storage phosphor, solid state detector.

inherent filtration: (see **filter**).

intraoral radiograph: Radiograph produced on an image receptor placed intraorally and lingually or palatally to the teeth.

in utero: In the uterus; refers to a fetus or embryo.

inverse square law: A physical law stating that in the absence of intervening absorbers, the intensity of radiation from a point source is inversely proportional to the square of the distance from the source. Example: A point source that produces 10 Gy h^{-1} at 1 m will produce 2.5 Gy h^{-1} at 2 m.

ionization chamber: A device for detection of ionizing radiation or for measurement of radiation exposure and exposure rate.

ionizing radiation: Any electromagnetic or particulate radiation capable of producing ions, directly or indirectly, by interaction with matter. Examples are x-ray photons, charged atomic particles and other ions, and neutrons.

kerma (*K*) (kinetic energy released per unit mass): The sum of the initial kinetic energies of all the charged particles liberated by uncharged particles per unit mass of a specified material. The SI unit for kerma is J kg^{-1} with the special name gray (Gy). 1 Gy = 1 J kg^{-1}. Kerma can be quoted for any specified material at a point in free space or in an absorbing medium (see also **air kerma**).

kilovolt (kV): A unit of electrical potential difference equal to 1,000 volts.

kilovolt peak (kVp): (also see **operating potential**). The crest value in kilovolts of the potential difference of a pulsating potential generator. When only one-half of the wave is used, the value refers to the useful half of the cycle. In this Report, the potential formed by a constant-potential generator is also expressed as kVp. In equations, in this Report, the symbol V_t is used, meaning the operating potential applied to the x-ray tube (*i.e.*, the kVp).

latent image: The invisible change produced in an x-ray or photographic film emulsion by the action of x radiation or light, from which the visible image is subsequently developed and fixed chemically; or the change produced in a photostimulable storage phosphor and recovered by scanning with a laser.

latitude: The range between the minimum and maximum radiation exposures to an image receptor that yield diagnostic images of structures.

leaded apron: An apron made with lead, a radiation absorbing material used to reduce radiation exposure.

leaded glove: A glove made with lead, a radiation absorbing material used to reduce radiation exposure.

lead equivalent: The thickness of lead affording the same attenuation, under specified conditions, as the material in question.

leakage radiation: (see **radiation**).

leakage technique factors: Technique factors specified for source assemblies at which leakage radiation is measured.

linear-energy transfer (LET): The linear rate of loss of energy by an ionizing photon or charged particle traversing a medium, usually reported in units of keV μm^{-1}.

low-LET: Particulate or electromagnetic radiation resulting in LET below approximately 10 keV μm^{-1}; electrons and x or gamma rays are common examples.

high-LET: Particulate radiation resulting in LET greater than about 10 to 100 keV μm^{-1}; neutrons and alpha particles are common examples.

magnification (in medical x-ray imaging): An imaging procedure carried out with magnification usually produced by purposeful introduction of distance between the subject and the image receptor.

material safety data sheet: Written or printed material concerning a hazardous chemical that is prepared in accordance with an Occupational Safety and Health Administration regulation (OSHA, 1994a).

milliampere (mA): Electrically, 1×10^{-3} ampere. In radiography, the current flow from the cathode to the anode that, in turn, regulates the intensity of radiation emitted by the x-ray tube, thus directly influencing radiographic density.

milliampere-minutes (mA min): The product of the x-ray tube operating current and exposure time, in minutes.

milliampere-seconds (mAs): The product of the x-ray tube operating current and exposure time, in seconds.

minimum detectable level: The threshold of detection for the device in question.

monitor: To determine the level of ionizing radiation or radioactive contamination in a given region. Also, a device used for this purpose.

multiple tube installation: An installation consisting of more than one x-ray source in the same room or of sources located in adjacent rooms that are close enough to require consideration of their combined workloads in radiation protection design.

natural background radiation: Radiation originating in natural sources: *e.g.*, cosmic rays, naturally occurring radioactive minerals, naturally occurring radioactive ^{14}C and ^{40}K in the body.

noise: The presence of random fluctuations in image intensity that do not relate to the subject being imaged. Noise is related to both speed and resolution. Generally, faster systems have greater noise.

occlusal radiograph: An intraoral radiograph made with the image receptor placed between the occlusal surfaces of the teeth, parallel to the occlusal plane, with the x-ray beam directed caudad or cephalad.

occupancy factor (*T*): The factor by which the workload should be multiplied to correct for the degree of occupancy (by any one person) of the area in question while the source is in the "ON" condition and emitting radiation. This multiplication is carried out for radiation protection purposes to determine compliance with shielding design goals.

occupational exposure: Exposures to individuals that are incurred in the workplace as a result of situations that can reasonably be regarded as being the responsibility of management (exposures associated with medical diagnosis or treatment for the individual are excluded).

operating potential: (also see **kilovolt peak**). The potential difference between the anode and cathode of an x-ray tube.

operator: Any individual who personally utilizes or manipulates a source of radiation.

optically-stimulated luminescent (OSL) dosimeter: A dosimeter containing a crystalline solid for measuring radiation dose, plus filters (absorbers) to help characterize the types of radiation encountered. When irradiated with intense light, OSL crystals that have been exposed to ionizing radiation give off light proportional to the energy they received from the radiation. The intense illuminating light needs to be of a different wavelength than the emitted light.

oral and maxillofacial radiology: The dental specialty that deals with the production and interpretation of images of dentomaxillofacial structures, practiced by a dental specialist who has undergone additional training in the use of imaging procedures for diagnosis and treatment of diseases, injuries, and abnormalities of the orofacial structures. In general, the individual should be credentialed by either the American Board of Oral and Maxillofacial Radiology or a comparable specialty board, or be eligible to sit for credentialing by such a board.

panoramic radiography (pantomography): A method of radiography by which continuous tomograms of the maxillary and mandibular dental arches and their associated structures may be obtained.

paralleling technique (parallel geometry): Intraoral radiography in which the plane of the image receptor is parallel to the long axes of the teeth being radiographed. The central beam of the x-ray field is directed at right angles to both.

periapical radiograph: An intraoral radiograph that demonstrates the crowns and roots of teeth and the surrounding alveolar bone structures.

personal dosimeter: A small radiation detector that is worn by an individual. Common personal dosimeters contain film, thermoluminescent or optically-stimulated luminescent materials as the radiation detection device.

personal protective equipment: Specialized clothing or equipment worn by an employee to protect against a hazard. General work clothes not intended to serve as protection against a hazard are not considered to be personal protective equipment.

phantom: An object used to simulate the absorption and scatter characteristics of the patient's body for radiation measurement purposes.

photon: A quantum of electromagnetic radiation.

pixel: A two-dimensional picture element in a digital image.

position-indicating device (PID) (cone, pointer cone, pointer): An open-ended device on a dental x-ray machine (in the shape of a cylinder or parallelepiped) designed to indicate the direction of the central ray and to serve as a guide in establishing a desired source-to-image receptor distance. Provision for beam collimation and added filtration can be incorporated into the construction of the device.

short cone: An open ended cylinder that establishes a source-to-image receptor distance of approximately 20 cm.

long cone: An open ended cylinder that establishes a source-to-image receptor distance of about 40 cm.

potentially exposed: In this Report, all monitored and unmonitored personnel who have the potential for being exposed to radiation in the course of their duties.

protective barrier: A barrier of radiation absorbing material(s) used to reduce radiation exposure.

primary protective barrier: A protective barrier used to attenuate the useful beam for radiation protection purposes.

secondary protective barrier: A barrier sufficient to attenuate scattered and leakage radiation for radiation protection purposes.

qualified expert: As used in this Report, a medical physicist or medical health physicist who is competent to design radiation shielding in dental x-ray facilities, and to advise regarding other radiation protection needs of dental x-ray installations. The qualified expert is a person who is certified by the American Board of Radiology, American Board of Medical Physicists, American Board of Health Physics, or Canadian College of Physicists in Medicine.

quality assurance: The mechanisms to ensure continuously optimal functioning of both technical and operational aspects of radiologic procedures to produce maximal diagnostic information while minimizing patient radiation exposure.

rad: The special name for the previous unit of absorbed dose. 1 rad = 0.01 J kg^{-1}. In the SI system of units, it is replaced by the special name gray (Gy). 1 Gy = 100 rad.

radiation (ionizing): Electromagnetic radiation (x or gamma rays) or particulate radiation (alpha particles, beta particles, electrons, positrons, protons, neutrons, and heavy charged particles) capable of producing ions by direct or secondary processes in passage through matter.

leakage radiation: All radiation coming from within the source assembly except for the useful beam. It includes the portion of the radiation coming directly from the source and not absorbed by the source assembly, as well as the scattered radiation produced within the source assembly.

scattered radiation: Radiation that, during interaction with matter, is changed in direction. The change is usually accompanied by a decrease in energy. For purposes of radiation protection, scattered radiation is assumed to come primarily from interactions of primary radiation with tissues of the patient.

useful beam: The radiation that passes through the opening in the beam-limiting device that is used for imaging.

radiation biology (radiobiology): That branch of science dealing with radiation effects on biological systems.

radiation protection survey: An evaluation of the radiation protection in and around an installation that includes radiation measurements, inspections, evaluations and recommendations.

radiation weighting factor (w_R): The factor by which the absorbed dose in a tissue or organ is modified to account for the type and energy of radiation in determining the probability of stochastic effects. For diagnostic x rays the radiation weighting factor is assigned the value of one.

radiograph: A film or other record produced by the action of x rays on a sensitized surface.

radiography: The production of images on film or other record by the action of x rays transmitted through the patient.

radiology: That branch of healing arts and sciences that deals with the use of images in the diagnosis and treatment of disease.

rare earth: Commonly used to refer to intensifying screens that contain one or more of the rare-earth elements and that make use of the absorption and conversion features of these elements in x-ray imaging.

receptor: Any device that absorbs a portion of the incident radiation energy and converts this portion into another form of energy that can be more easily used to produce desired results (*e.g.*, production of an image) (also see **image receptor**).

regulated medical waste: Regulated medical waste consists of: (1) liquid or semi-liquid blood or other potentially infectious materials, (2) contaminated items that would release blood or other potentially infectious materials in a liquid or semi-liquid state when compressed, (3) items caked with dried blood or other potentially infectious materials and capable of releasing these materials when handled, (4) contaminated sharps, and (5) pathological and microbiological wastes containing blood or other potentially infectious materials.

relative risk: The ratio of the risk of a given disease in those exposed to the risk of that disease in those not exposed.

excess relative risk: Relative risk minus one (*i.e.*, the fractional increase in incidence in the irradiated population).

rem: The special name for the previous unit numerically equal to the absorbed dose (D) in rad, modified by a quality factor (Q). 1 rem = 0.01 J kg^{-1}. In the SI system of units, it is replaced by the special name sievert (Sv), which is numerically equal to the absorbed dose (D) in gray modified by a radiation weighting factor (w_R). 1 Sv = 100 rem.

resolution: In the context of an image system, the output of which is finally viewed by the eye, it refers to the smallest size or highest spatial frequency of an object of given contrast that is just perceptible. The intrinsic resolution, or resolving power, of an imaging system is measured in line pairs per millimeter (lp mm^{-1}), ordinarily using a resolving power target. The resolution actually achieved when imaging lower contrast objects is normally much less, and depends upon many variables such as subject contrast levels and noise of the overall imaging system.

roentgen (R): The special name for exposure, which is a specific quantity of ionization (charge) produced by the absorption of x- or gamma-radiation energy in a specified mass of air under standard conditions. 1 R = 2.58×10^{-4} coulombs per kilogram (C kg^{-1}).

safelight: Special lighting used in a darkroom that permits film to be transferred from cassette to processor without fogging.

scatter: Deflection of radiation interacting with matter, causing change of direction of subatomic particles or photons, attenuation of the radiation beam, and usually some absorption of energy.

scattered radiation: (see **radiation**).

secondary protective barrier: (see **protective barrier**).

sharpness (image): (see **resolution**).

shielding design goals (*P*): Practical radiation levels, measured at a reference point beyond a protective barrier, that result in the respective annual effective dose limit for workers or the general public not being exceeded, when combined with conservatively safe assumptions in the structural shielding design calculations. For low-LET radiation, the quantity air kerma is used. P can be expressed as an annual or weekly value (*e.g.*, mGy $week^{-1}$ or mGy y^{-1} air kerma).

sievert (Sv): The special name for the SI unit of dose equivalent (H), equivalent dose (H_T) and effective dose (E). 1 Sv = 1 J kg^{-1}.

signal-to-noise ratio: The ratio of input signal to background interference. The greater the ratio, the clearer the image.

source assembly: (see **diagnostic source assembly**).

source-to-image receptor distance: The distance, measured along the central ray, from the center of the front surface of the source (x-ray focal spot) to the surface of the image receptor.

source-to-surface distance (source-to-skin distance): The distance, measured along the central ray, from the center of the front surface of the source (x-ray focal spot) to the surface of the irradiated object or patient.

spatial resolution: (see **resolution**).

speed: (also see **film speed**). As applied to an image receptor, an index of the relative exposure required to produce an image of acceptable quality; faster image receptors need less exposure.

stepwedge: A device consisting of increments of an absorber through which a radiographic exposure is made on film to permit determination of the amounts of radiation reaching the film by measurements of film density.

stochastic effects: Effects, the probability of which, rather than their severity, is a function of radiation dose, implying the absence of a threshold. (More generally, stochastic means random in nature).

survey meter: An instrument or device, usually portable, for monitoring the level of radiation or of radioactive contamination in an area or location.

target: The part of an x-ray tube anode assembly impacted by the electron beam to produce the useful x-ray beam.

thermoluminescent dosimeter: A dosimeter containing a crystalline solid for measuring radiation dose, plus filters (absorbers) to help characterize the types of radiation encountered. When heated, thermoluminescent dosimeter crystals that have been exposed to ionizing radiation give off light proportional to the energy they received from the radiation.

tissue weighting factor (w_T): The factor by which the equivalent dose in tissue or organ T is weighted, and which represents the relative contribution of that organ or tissue to the total detriment due to stochastic effects resulting from uniform irradiation of the whole body.

tomography: A special technique to show in detail images of structures lying in a predetermined plane of tissue, while blurring or eliminating detail in images of structures in other planes.

universal precautions: An approach to infection control in which all human blood and certain human body fluids are treated as if known to be infectious for human immunodeficiency virus, hepatitis B virus, and other blood-borne pathogens. Other potentially infectious materials include semen, vaginal secretions, cerebrospinal fluid, peritoneal fluid, amniotic fluid, saliva, any body fluid that is visibly contaminated with blood, and all body fluids in situations where it is difficult or impossible to differentiate between body fluids.

use factor (*U*): Fraction of the workload during which the useful beam is directed at the barrier under consideration.

useful beam: (see **radiation**).

user: Dentists, physicians and others responsible for the radiation exposure of patients.

waveform: An expression of the temporal variation of the operating potential applied to the x-ray tube in the course of an exposure.

single-phase: Produced by conventional alternating current line current.

half-wave rectified: Producing a single 1/120 s pulse of x rays during each 1/60 s alternating current cycle.

full-wave rectified: Producing two 1/120 s pulses of x rays during each 1/60 s alternating current cycle.

three-phase: Produced by three-phase full-wave rectified current, providing 12 overlapping 1/120 s pulses during each 1/60 s alternating current cycle.

constant potential: Produced by electronic manipulation of alternating line current to provide constant tube voltage and a beam energy spectrum that varies little or not at all during exposure.

workload (*W*): The degree of use of a radiation source. For the dental x-ray machines covered in this Report, the workload is expressed in milliampere-minutes per week (mA min $week^{-1}$).

x rays: Electromagnetic radiation typically produced by high-energy electrons impinging on a metal target.

References

AADR (1983). American Academy of Dental Radiology. "Recommendations for quality assurance in dental radiography," Oral Surg. Oral Med. Oral Pathol. **55**(4), 421–426.

ADA (1970). American Dental Association. "Revised American Dental Association Specification No. 22 for intraoral dental radiographic film," J. Am. Dent. Assoc. **80**(5), 1066–1068.

ADA (1989). American Dental Association. "Recommendations in radiographic practices: An update, 1988," J. Am. Dent. Assoc. **118**(1), 115–117.

ADA (1996). American Dental Association. "Infection control recommendations for the dental office and the dental laboratory," J. Am. Dent. Assoc. **127**(5), 672–680.

ANSI (1996). American National Standards Institute. *Photography—Intra-Oral Dental Radiographic Film—Specification,* ANSI/ISO 3665 (American National Standards Institute, New York).

ARCHER, B.R., THORNBY, J.I. and BUSHONG, S.C. (1983). "Diagnostic x-ray shielding design based on an empirical model of photon attenuation," Health Phys. **44**, 507–517.

ARCHER, B.R., FEWELL, T.R., CONWAY, B.J. and QUINN, P.W. (1994). "Attenuation properties of diagnostic x-ray shielding materials," Med. Phys. **21**(9), 1499–1507.

AROUA, A., BURNAND, B., DECKA, I., VADER, J.P. and VALLEY, J.F. (2002). "Nation-wide survey on radiation doses in diagnostic and interventional radiology in Switzerland in 1998," Health Phys. **83**, 46–55.

ATCHISON, K.A., WHITE, S.C., FLACK, V.F. and HEWLETT, E.R. (1995). "Assessing the FDA guidelines for ordering dental radiographs," J. Am. Dent. Assoc. **126**(10), 1372–1383.

AVENDANIO, B., FREDERIKSEN, N.L., BENSON, B.W. and SOKOLOWSKI, T.W. (1996). "Effective dose and risk assessment from detailed narrow beam radiography," Oral Surg. Oral Med. Oral Pathol. Oral Radiol. Endod. **82**(6), 713–719.

BITHELL, J.F. (1989). "Epidemiological studies of children irradiated *in utero*," pages 77 to 87 in *Low-Dose Radiation: Biological Bases of Risk Assessment*, Baverstock, K.F. and Stather, J.W., Eds. (Taylor and Francis, New York).

BOHAY, R.N., STEPHENS, R.G. and KOGON, S.L. (1995a). "Radiographic examination of children. A survey of prescribing practices of general dentists," Oral Surg. Oral Med. Oral Pathol. Oral Radiol. Endod. **79**(5), 641–645.

BOHAY, R.N., STEPHENS, R.G. and KOGON, S.L. (1995b). "Survey of radiographic practices of general dentists for the dentate adult patient," Oral Surg. Oral Med. Oral Pathol. Oral Radiol. Endod. **79**(4), 526–531.

BOHAY, R.N., STEPHENS, R.G. and KOGON, S.L. (1998). "A study of the impact of screening or selective radiography on the treatment and postdelivery outcome for edentulous patients," Oral Surg. Oral Med. Oral Pathol. Oral Radiol. Endod. **86**(3), 353–359.

BOICE, J.D., JR., LAND, C.E. and PRESTON, D.L. (1996). "Ionizing radiation," pages 319 to 354 in *Cancer Epidemiology and Prevention*, Schottenfeld, D. and Fraumeni, J.F. Jr., Eds. (Oxford University Press, New York).

BOICE, J.D., JR. and MILLER, R.W. (1999). "Childhood and adult cancer after intrauterine exposure to ionizing radiation," Teratology **59**, 227–233.

BRAND, J., BENSON, B., CIOLA, B., GLASS, B., KATZ, J., OTIS, L. and PARKS, E. (1992). "American Academy of Oral and Maxillofacial Radiology infection control guidelines for dental radiographic procedures," Oral Surg. Oral Med. Oral Pathol. **73**(2), 248–249.

BRENNER, D.J., DOLL. R., GOODHEAD, D.T., HALL, E.J., LAND, C.E., LITTLE, J.B., LUBIN, J.H., PRESTON, D.L., PRESTON, R.J., PUSKIN, J.S., RON, E., SACHS, R.K., SAMET, J.M., SETLOW, R.B. and ZAIDER, M. (2003). "Cancer risks attributable to low doses of ionizing radiation: Assessing what we really know," Proc. Natl. Acad. Sci. USA **100**, 13761–13766.

BRENT, R.L. (1999). "Utilization of developmental basic science principles in the evaluation of reproductive risks from pre- and postconception environmental radiation exposures," Teratology **59**(4), 182–204.

BROOKS, S.L. (1986). "A study of selection criteria for intraoral dental radiography," Oral Surg. Oral Med. Oral Pathol. **62**(2), 234–239.

BROOKS, S.L. and CHO, S.Y. (1993). "Validation of a specific selection criterion for dental periapical radiography," Oral Surg. Oral Med. Oral Pathol. **75**(3), 383–386.

BROWN, R.J., SHAVER, J.W. and LAMEL, D.A. (1980). *The Selection of Patients for X-Ray Examinations*, HEW Publication FDA 80-8104 (Center for Devices and Radiological Health, Rockville, Maryland).

BUDOWSKY, J., PIRO, J.D., ZEGARELLI, E.V., KUTSCHER, A.H. and BARNETT, A. (1956). "Radiation exposure to the head and abdomen during oral roentgenography," J. Am. Dent. Assoc. **52**(5), 555–559.

BURCH, J.D., CRAIB, K.J., CHOI, B.C., MILLER, A.B., RISCH, H.A. and HOWE, G.R. (1987). "An exploratory case-control study of brain tumors in adults," J. Natl. Cancer Inst. **78**(4), 601–609.

BUSHBERG, J.T., SEIBERT, J.A., LEIDHOLDT, E.M., JR. and BOONE, J.M. (2001). *The Essential Physics of Medical Imaging*, 2nd ed. (Lippincott Williams and Wilkins, Baltimore, Maryland).

CALLEN, T. (1994). "A comparative study of the selection criteria and diagnostic yield in panoramic radiography for patients attending

Manchester and Indianapolis dental hospitals," Pro. Br. Soc. Dent. Maxillofac. Radiol. **6**, 24–36.

CDC (2003). Centers for Disease Control and Prevention. *Guidelines for Infection Control in Dental Health-Care Settings*, MMWR 52 (RR-17) (Centers for Disease Control and Prevention, Atlanta, Georgia).

CEDERBURG, R.A., FREDERIKSEN, N.L., BENSON, B.W. and SOKOLOWSKI, T.W. (1997). "Effect of the geometry of the intraoral position-indicating device on effective dose," Oral Surg. Oral Med. Oral Pathol. Oral Radiol. Endod. **84**(1), 101–109.

COHEN, B.L. (2002). "Cancer risk from low-level radiation," Am. J. Roentgenol. **179**, 1137–1143.

CONOVER, G.L., HILDEBOLT, C.F. and ANTHONY, D. (1995). "Objective and subjective evaluations of Kodak Ektaspeed Plus dental x-ray film," Oral Surg. Oral Med. Oral Pathol. Oral Radiol. Endod. **79**(2), 246–250.

CRCPD (2003). Conference of Radiation Control Program Directors, Inc. *Patient Exposure and Dose Guide–2003*, CRCPD Publication E-03-2 (Conference of Radiation Control Program Directors, Inc., Frankfort, Kentucky).

D'AMBROSIO, J.A., SCHIFF, T.G., MCDAVID, W.D. and LANGLAND, O.E. (1986). "Diagnostic quality versus patient exposure with five panoramic screen-film combinations," Oral Surg. Oral Med. Oral Pathol. **61**(4), 409–411.

DAVIS, F.G., BOICE, J.D., JR., KELSEY, J.L. and MONSON, R.R. (1987). "Cancer mortality after multiple fluoroscopic examinations of the chest," J. Natl. Cancer Inst. **78**(4), 645–652.

DE HAAN, R.A. and VAN AKEN, J. (1990). "Effective dose equivalent to the operator in intra-oral dental radiography," Dentomaxillofac. Radiol. **19**(3), 113–118.

DELONGCHAMP, R.R., MABUCHI, K., YOSHIMOTO Y. and PRESTON, D.L. (1997). "Cancer mortality among atomic bomb survivors exposed *in utero* or as young children, October 1950-May 1992," Radiat. Res. **147**, 385–395.

DIEHL, R., GRATT, B.M. and GOULD, R.G. (1986). "Radiographic quality control measurements comparing D-speed film, E-speed film, and xeroradiography," Oral Surg. Oral Med. Oral Pathol. **61**(6), 635–640.

DIXON, R.L. and SIMPKIN, D.J. (1998). "Primary shielding barriers for diagnostic x-ray facilities: A new model," Health Phys. **74**(2), 181–189.

DOLL, R. and WAKEFORD, R. (1997). "Risk of childhood cancer from fetal irradiation," Br. J. Radiol. **70**, 130–139.

DUNN, S.M. and KANTOR, M.L. (1993). "Digital radiology. Facts and fictions," J. Am. Dent. Assoc. **124**(12), 38–47.

ELLIS, R.E. (1961). "The distribution of active bone marrow in the adult," Phys. Med. Biol. **5**, 255–258.

EPA (1986). U.S. Environmental Protection Agency. *EPA Guide for Infections Waste Management*, EPA/530-SW-86-014 (U.S. Environmental Protection Agency, Washington).

EPA (1990). U.S. Environmental Protection Agency. *Guides to Pollution Prevention: Selected Hospital Waste Streams,* EPA/625/7-90/009 (National Technical Information Service, Springfield, Virginia).

EPA (1994). U.S. Environmental Protection Agency. *Protection of the Environment. Subchapter 1. Solid Wastes,* 40 CFR (U.S. Government Printing Office, Washington).

FDA (1973). Food and Drug Administration. *Population Exposure to X-Rays: U.S. 1970: A Report on the Public Health Service X-Ray Exposure Study,* U.S. HEW Publication (FDA) 73-8047 (U.S. Government Printing Office, Washington).

FDA (1995). Food and Drug Administration. *Performance Standards for Ionizing Radiation Emitting Products,* 21 CFR 1020 (U.S. Government Printing Office, Washington).

FARMAN, T.T. and FARMAN, A.G. (2000). "Evaluation of a new F speed dental x-ray film. The effect of processing solutions and a comparison with D and E speeds films." Dentomaxillofac. Radiol. **29**(1), 41–45.

FLINT, D.J., PAUNOVICH, E., MOORE, W.S., WOFFORD, D.T. and HERMESCH, C.B. (1998). "A diagnostic comparison of panoramic and intraoral radiographs," Oral Surg. Oral Med. Oral Pathol. Oral Radiol. Endod. **85**(6), 731–735.

FREEDMAN, M.L. and MATTESON, S.R. (1976). "A collimator for reduced radiation dose with improved visualization of soft tissues," Radiology **118**(1), 226–228.

FREEMAN, J.P. and BRAND, J.W. (1994). "Radiation doses of commonly used dental radiographic surveys," Oral Surg. Oral Med. Oral Pathol. **77**(3), 285–289.

FRIEDLAND, B. (1998). "Clinical radiological issues in orthodontic practice," Semin. Orthod. **4**(2), 64–78.

FROMMER, H.H. and JAIN, R.K. (1987). "A comparative clinical study of group D and E dental film," Oral Surg. Oral Med. Oral Pathol. **63**(6), 738–742.

FURKART, A.J., DOVE, S.B., MCDAVID, W.D., NUMMIKOSKI, P. and MATTESON, S. (1992). "Direct digital radiography for the detection of periodontal bone lesions," Oral Surg. Oral Med. Oral Pathol. **74**(5), 652–660.

GARDNER, M.J., SNEE, M.P., HALL, A.J., POWELL, C.A., DOWNES, S. and TERRELL, J.D. (1990). "Results of case-control study of leukaemia and lymphoma among young people near Sellafield nuclear plant in West Cumbria," Br. Med. J. **300**(6722), 423–429.

GIBBS, S.J. (1989). "Influence of organs in the ICRP's remainder on effective dose equivalent computed for diagnostic radiation exposures," Health Phys. **56**(4), 515–520.

GIBBS, S.J. (2000). "Effective dose equivalent and effective dose: Comparison for common projections in oral and maxillofacial radiology," Oral Surg. Oral Med. Oral Pathol. Oral Radiol. Endod. **90**(4), 538–545.

GIBBS, S.J., PUJOL, A., JR., CHEN, T.S., CARLTON, J.C., DOSMANN, M.A., MALCOLM, A.W. and JAMES, A.E., JR. (1987). "Radiation doses to sensitive organs from intraoral dental radiography," Dentomaxillofac. Radiol. **16**(2), 67–77.

GIBBS, S.J., PUJOL, A., JR., CHEN, T.S. and JAMES, A.E., JR. (1988a). "Patient risk from intraoral dental radiography," Dentomaxillofac. Radiol. **17**(1), 15–23.

GIBBS, S.J., PUJOL, A., MCDAVID, W.D., WELANDER, U. and TRONJE, G. (1988b). "Patient risk from rotational panoramic radiography," Dentomaxillofac. Radiol. **17**(1), 25–32.

GILBERT, E.S., TARONE, R., BOUVILLE, A. and RON, E. (1998). "Thyroid cancer rates and ^{131}I doses from Nevada atmospheric nuclear bomb tests," J. Natl. Cancer Inst. **90**, 1654–1660.

GILES, D., HEWITT, D., STEWART, A. and WEBB, J. (1956). "Malignant disease in childhood and diagnostic irradiation *in utero*," Lancet **271**, 447.

GOREN, A.D., SCIUBBA, J.J., FRIEDMAN, R. and MALAMUD, H. (1989). "Survey of radiologic practices among dental practitioners," Oral Surg. Oral Med. Oral Pathol. **67**(4), 464–468.

GRAHAM, S., LEVIN, M.L., LILIENFELD, A.M., SCHUMAN, L.M., GIBSON, R., DOWD, J.E. and HEMPELMANN, L. (1966). "Preconception, intrauterine, and postnatal irradiation as related to leukemia," Natl. Cancer Inst. Monogr. **19**, 347–371.

GRATT, B.M., WHITE, S.C., PACKARD, F.L. and PETERSSON, A.R. (1984). "An evaluation of rare-earth imaging systems in panoramic radiography," Oral Surg. Oral Med. Oral Pathol. **58**(4), 475–482.

GRAY, J.E., ARCHER, B.R., BUTLER, P., HOBBS, B.B., METTLER, F., PIZZUTIELLO, R., JR, SCHUELER, B.A., STRAUSS, M.S., SULEIMAN, O. and YAFFE, M. (in press). "Reference values for diagnostic Radiology: Application and impact," Radiology.

HALL, E.J. (1994). *Radiobiology for the Radiologist*, 4th ed. (Lippincott, Philadelphia).

HALL, P., MATTSSON, A. and BOICE, J.D., JR. (1996). "Thyroid cancer after diagnostic administration of ^{131}I," Radiat. Res. **145**, 86–92.

HEMPELMANN, L.H., HALL, W.J., PHILLIPS, M., COOPER, R.A. and AMES, W.R. (1975). "Neoplasms in persons treated with x-rays in infancy: Fourth survey in 20 years," J. Natl. Cancer Inst. **55**(3), 519–530.

HINTZE, H., WENZEL, A. and JONES, C. (1994). "*In vitro* comparison of D- and E-speed film radiography, RVG, and Visualix digital radiography for the detection of enamel approximal and dentinal occlusal caries lesions," Caries Res. **28**(5), 363–367.

HINTZE, H., CHRISTOFFERSEN, L. and WENZEL, A. (1996). "*In vitro* comparison of Kodak Ultra-Speed, Ektaspeed, and Ektaspeed Plus, and Agfa M2 Comfort dental x-ray films for the detection of caries," Oral Surg. Oral Med. Oral Pathol. Oral Radiol. Endod. **81**(2), 240–244.

HSE (1998). Health and Safety Executive. *Occupational Exposure to Ionizing Radiation: Analysis of Doses Reported to the Health and Safety*

Executive's Central Index of Dose Information (Her Majesty's Stationery Office, Norwich, United Kingdom).

ICRP (1977). International Commission on Radiological Protection. *Recommendations of the International Commission on Radiological Protection*, ICRP Publication 26, Annals of the ICRP **1**(3) (Elsevier Science, New York).

ICRP (1988). International Commission on Radiological Protection. *Data for Use in Protection Against External Radiation*, ICRP Publication 51, Annuals of the ICRP **17**(2/3) (Elsevier Science, New York).

ICRP (1991). International Commission on Radiological Protection. *1990 Recommendations of the International Commission on Radiological Protection*, ICRP Publication 60, Annals of the ICRP **21**(1-3) (Elsevier Science, New York).

ICRP (1993). International Commission on Radiological Protection. "Summary of current ICRP principles for protection of the patient in diagnostic radiology," in *Radiological Protection in Biomedical Research*, ICRP Publication 62, Annals of the ICRP **22**(3) (Elsevier Science, New York).

ICRP (1996a). International Commission on Radiological Protection. *Radiological Protection and Safety in Medicine*, ICRP Publication 73, Annals of the ICRP **26**(2) (Elsevier Science, New York).

ICRP (1996b). International Commission on Radiological Protection. *Conversion Coefficients for Use in Radiological Protection Against External Radiation*, ICRP Publication 74, Annals of the ICRP **26**(3-4) (Elsevier Science, New York).

ICRU (1993). International Commission on Radiation Units and Measurements. *Quantities and Units in Radiation Protection Dosimetry*, ICRU Report 51 (International Commission on Radiation Units and Measurements, Bethesda, Maryland).

ICRU (1998). International Commission on Radiation Units and Measurements. *Fundamental Quantities and Units for Ionizing Radiation*, ICRU Report 60 (International Commission on Radiation Units and Measurements, Bethesda, Maryland).

IEC (1994). International Electrotechnical Commission. *Medical Electrical Equipment - Part 1: General Requirements for Safety - 3. Collateral Standard: General Requirements for Radiation Protection in Diagnostic X-Ray Equipment*, SS-EN 60601-1-3 (International Electrotechnical Commission, Geneva).

JABLON, S. and KATO, H. (1970). "Childhood cancer in relation to prenatal exposure to atomic-bomb radiation," Lancet **2**(7681), 1000–1003.

JACOB, P., KENIGSBERG, Y., ZVONOVA, I., GOULKO, G., BUGLOVA, E., HEIDENREICH, W.F., GOLOVNEVA, A., BRATILOVA, A.A., DROZDOVITCH, V., KRUK, J., POCHTENNAJA, G.T., BALONOV, M., DEMIDCHIK, E.P. and PARETZKE, H.G. (1999). "Childhood exposure due to the Chernobyl accident and thyroid cancer risk in contaminated areas of Belarus and Russia," Br. J. Cancer **80**, 1461–1469.

JACOBI, W. (1975). "The concept of the effective dose—a proposal for the combination of organ doses," Radiat. Environ. Biophys. **12**(2), 101–109.

JOHNS, H.E. and CUNNINGHAM, J.R. (1983). *The Physics of Radiology* (Charles C. Thomas, Springfield, Illinois).

JOSEPH, L. (1987). *Selection of Patients for X-Ray Examinations: Dental Radiographic Examinations*, HHS Publication FDA 88-8273 (U.S. Department of Health and Human Services, Rockville, Maryland).

KARLSSON, P., HOLMBERG, E., LUNDELL, M., MATTSSON, A., HOLM, L.E. and WALLGREN, A. (1998). "Intracranial tumors after exposure to ionizing radiation during infancy: A pooled analysis of two Swedish cohorts of 28,008 infants with skin hemangioma," Radiat. Res. **150,** 357–364.

KAUGARS, G.E. and FATOUROS, P. (1982). "Clinical comparison of conventional and rare earth screen-film systems for cephalometric radiographs," Oral Surg. Oral Med. Oral Pathol. **53**, 322–325.

KAUL, A., LANDFERMANN, H. and THIEME, M. (1996). "One decade after Chernobyl: Summing up the consequences," Health Phys. **71**(5), 634–640.

KITAGAWA, H., FARMAN, A.G., WAKOH, M., NISHIKAWA, K. and KUROYANAGI, K. (1995). "Objective and subjective assessments of Kodak Ektaspeed plus new dental x-ray film: A comparison with other conventional x-ray films," Bull. Tokyo Dent. Coll. **36**(2), 61–67.

KLEIER, D.J., HICKS, M.J. and FLAITZ, C.M. (1987). "A comparison of Ultraspeed and Ektaspeed dental x-ray film: *In vitro* study of the radiographic appearance of interproximal lesions," Oral Surg. Oral Med. Oral Pathol. **63**(3), 381–385.

KODAK (1991). Eastman Kodak Company. *Management of Photographic Wastes in the Dental Office, Kodak Dental Radiography Series*, Publication No. N-417 (Eastman Kodak Company, Rochester, New York).

KOGON, S., BOHAY, R. and STEPHENS, R. (1995). "A survey of the radiographic practices of general dentists for edentulous patients," Oral Surg. Oral Med. Oral Pathol. Oral Radiol. Endod. **80**(3), 365–368.

KULLENDORF, F.B., NILSSON, M. and ROHLIN, M. (1996). "Diagnostic accuracy of direct digital dental radiography for the detection of periapical bone lesions: Overall comparison between conventional and direct digital radiography," Oral Surg. Oral Med. Oral Pathol. Oral Radiol. Endod. **82**(3), 344–350.

KUMAZAWA, S., NELSON, D.R. and RICHARDSON, A.C.B. (1984). *Occupational Exposure to Ionizing Radiation in the United States: A Comprehensive Review for the Year 1980 and a Summary of Trends for the Years 1960-1985*, EPA 520/1-84/005 (National Technical Information Service, Springfield, Virginia).

LAWS, P.W. and ROSENSTEIN, M. (1978). "A somatic dose index for diagnostic radiology," Health Phys. **35**(5), 629–642.

LIVSHITS, L.A., MALYARCHUK, S.G., LUKYANOVA, E.M., ANTIPKIN, Y.G., ARABSKAYA, L.P., KRAVCHENKO, S.A., MATSUKA, G.H.,

PETIT, E., GIRAUDEAU, F., GOURMELON, P., VERGNAUD, G. and LE GUEN, B. (2001). "Children of Chernobyl cleanup workers do not show elevated rates of mutations in minisatellite alleles," Radiat. Res. **155**, 74–80.

LUDLOW, J.B. and PLATIN, E. (1995). "Densitometric comparisons of Ultra-speed, Ektaspeed, and Ektaspeed Plus intraoral films for two processing conditions," Oral Surg. Oral Med. Oral Pathol. Oral Radiol. Endod. **79**(1), 105–113.

LUDLOW, J.B., ABREU, M., JR. and MOL, A. (2001). "Performance of a new F-speed film for caries detection," Dentomaxillofac. Radiol. **30**(2), 110–113.

MACDONALD, J.C., REID, J.A. and BERTHOTY, D. (1983). "Drywall construction as a dental radiation barrier," Oral Surg. Oral Med. Oral Pathol. **55**(3), 319–326.

MALKIN, J. (2002). *Medical and Dental Space Planning: A Comprehensive Guide to Design, Equipment, and Clinical Procedures*, 3rd ed. (John Wiley & Sons, New York).

MATTESON, S.R. (1997). "Radiographic guidelines for edentulous patients," Oral Surg. Oral Med. Oral Pathol. Oral Radiol. Endod. **83**(5), 624–626.

MATTESON, S.R., MORRISON, W.S., STANEK, E.J., III and PHILLIPS, C. (1983). "A survey of radiographs obtained at the initial dental examination and patient selection criteria for bitewings at recall," J. Am. Dent. Assoc. **107**(4), 586–590.

MATTESON, S.R., JOSEPH, L.P., BOTTOMLEY, W., FINGER, H.W., FROMMER, H.H., KOCH, R.W., MATRANGA, L.F., NOWAK, A.J., RACHLIN, J.A., SCHOENFELD, C.M. *et al.* (1991). "The report of the panel to develop radiographic selection criteria for dental patients," Gen. Dent. **39**(4), 264–270.

METTLER, F.A., JR. (1987). "Diagnostic radiology: Usage and trends in the United States, 1964-1980," Radiology **162**, 263–266.

METTLER, F.A. and UPTON, A.C. (1995). *Medical Effects of Ionizing Radiation*, 2nd ed. (W. B. Saunders Co., Philadelphia).

MICHEL, R. and ZIMMERMAN, T.L. (1999). "Basic radiation protection considerations in dental practice," Health Phys. **77**(5), S81–83.

MODAN, B., RON, E. and WERNER, A. (1977). "Thyroid cancer following scalp irradiation," Radiology **123**(3), 741–744.

NAKFOOR, C.A. and BROOKS, S.L. (1992). "Compliance of Michigan dentists with radiographic safety recommendations," Oral Surg. Oral Med. Oral Pathol. **73**(4), 510–513.

NAPIER, I.D. (1999). "Reference doses for dental radiography," Br. Dent. J. **186**(8), 392–396.

NAS/NRC (1990). National Academy of Sciences/National Research Council. *Health Effects of Exposure to Low Levels of Ionizing Radiation*, Committee on the Biological Effects of Ionizing Radiation (BEIR V) (National Academy Press, Washington).

NCHCT (1981). National Center for Health Care Technology. "Dental radiology: A summary of recommendations from the Technology Assessment Forum," J. Am. Dent. Assoc. **103**(3), 423–425.

NCHCT (1982). National Center for Health Care Technology. *Technology Assessment Forum on Dental Radiology*, HHS Publication FDA 82–8197 (U.S. Department of Health and Human Services, Rockville, Maryland).

NCRP (1966). National Council on Radiation Protection and Measurements. *Radiation Protection in Educational Institutions*, NCRP Report No. 32 (National Council on Radiation Protection and Measurements, Bethesda, Maryland).

NCRP (1970). National Council on Radiation Protection and Measurements. *Dental X-Ray Protection*, NCRP Report No. 35 (National Council on Radiation Protection and Measurements, Bethesda, Maryland).

NCRP (1976). National Council on Radiation Protection and Measurements. *Structural Shielding Design and Evaluation for Medical Use of X Rays and Gamma Rays of Energies up to 10 MeV*, NCRP Report No. 49 (National Council on Radiation Protection and Measurements, Bethesda, Maryland).

NCRP (1977). National Council on Radiation Protection and Measurements. *Medical Radiation Exposure of Pregnant and Potentially Pregnant Women*, NCRP Report No. 54 (National Council on Radiation Protection and Measurements, Bethesda, Maryland).

NCRP (1978). National Council on Radiation Protection and Measurements. *Instrumentation and Monitoring Methods for Radiation Protection*, NCRP Report No. 57 (National Council on Radiation Protection and Measurements, Bethesda, Maryland).

NCRP (1985). National Council on Radiation Protection and Measurements. *SI Units in Radiation Protection and Measurements*, NCRP Report No. 82 (National Council on Radiation Protection and Measurements, Bethesda, Maryland).

NCRP (1987a). National Council on Radiation Protection and Measurements. *Exposure of the Population in the United States and Canada from Natural Background Radiation*, NCRP Report No. 94 (National Council on Radiation Protection and Measurements, Bethesda, Maryland).

NCRP (1987b). National Council on Radiation Protection and Measurements. *Ionizing Radiation Exposure of the Population of the United States*, NCRP Report No. 93 (National Council on Radiation Protection and Measurements, Bethesda, Maryland).

NCRP (1987c). National Council on Radiation Protection and Measurements. *Radiation Exposure of the U.S. Population from Consumer Products and Miscellaneous Sources*, NCRP Report No. 95 (National Council on Radiation Protection and Measurements, Bethesda, Maryland).

NCRP (1988). National Council on Radiation Protection and Measurements. *Quality Assurance for Diagnostic Imaging*, NCRP Report

No. 99 (National Council on Radiation Protection and Measurements, Bethesda, Maryland).

NCRP (1989a). National Council on Radiation Protection and Measurements. *Medical X-Ray, Electron Beam and Gamma-Ray Protection for Energies Up to 50 MeV (Equipment Design, Performance and Use)*, NCRP Report No. 102 (National Council on Radiation Protection and Measurements, Bethesda, Maryland).

NCRP (1989b). National Council on Radiation Protection and Measurements. *Radiation Protection for Medical and Allied Health Personnel*, NCRP Report No. 105 (National Council on Radiation Protection and Measurements, Bethesda, Maryland).

NCRP (1989c). National Council on Radiation Protection and Measurements. *Exposure of the U.S. Population from Diagnostic Medical Radiation*, NCRP Report No. 100 (National Council on Radiation Protection and Measurements, Bethesda, Maryland).

NCRP (1989d). National Council on Radiation Protection and Measurements. *Exposure of the U.S. Population from Occupational Radiation*, NCRP Report No. 101 (National Council on Radiation Protection and Measurements, Bethesda, Maryland).

NCRP (1990). National Council on Radiation Protection and Measurements. *Implementation of the Principle of As Low as Reasonably Achievable (ALARA) for Medical and Dental Personnel*, NCRP Report No. 107 (National Council on Radiation Protection and Measurements, Bethesda, Maryland).

NCRP (1992). National Council on Radiation Protection and Measurements. *Maintaining Radiation Protection Records*, NCRP Report No. 114 (National Council on Radiation Protection and Measurements, Bethesda, Maryland).

NCRP (1993a). National Council on Radiation Protection and Measurements. *Limitation of Exposure to Ionizing Radiation*, NCRP Report No. 116 (National Council on Radiation Protection and Measurements, Bethesda, Maryland).

NCRP (1993b). National Council on Radiation Protection and Measurements. *Risk Estimates for Radiation Protection*, NCRP Report No. 115 (National Council on Radiation Protection and Measurements, Bethesda, Maryland).

NCRP (1997). National Council on Radiation Protection and Measurements. *Uncertainties in Fatal Cancer Risk Estimates Used in Radiation Protection*, NCRP Report No. 126 (National Council on Radiation Protection and Measurements, Bethesda, Maryland).

NCRP (1998). National Council on Radiation Protection and Measurements. *Operational Radiation Safety Program*, NCRP Report No. 127 (National Council on Radiation Protection and Measurements, Bethesda, Maryland).

NCRP (2000). National Council on Radiation Protection and Measurements. *Operational Radiation Safety Training*, NCRP Report No. 134

(National Council on Radiation Protection and Measurements, Bethesda, Maryland).

NCRP (2001). National Council on Radiation Protection and Measurements. *Evaluation of the Linear-Nonthreshold Dose-Response Model for Ionizing Radiation*, NCRP Report No. 136 (National Council on Radiation Protection and Measurements, Bethesda, Maryland).

NCRP (in press). National Council on Radiation Protection and Measurements. *Structural Shielding Design for Medical X-Ray Imaging Facilities*, NCRP Report No. 146 (National Council on Radiation Protection and Measurements, Bethesda, Maryland).

NRPB (1994). National Radiological Protection Board. *Guidelines on Radiology Standards for Primary Dental Care: Report by the Royal College of Radiologists and the National Radiological Protection Board*, Documents of the NRPB **5**(3) (National Radiation Protection Board, Chilton, United Kingdom).

NRPB (1999). National Radiological Protection Board. *Guidelines on Patient Dose to Promote the Optimisation of Protection for Diagnostic Medical Exposures: Report of an Advisory Group on Ionizing Radiation*, Documents of the NRPB **10**(1) (National Radiation Protection Board, Chilton, United Kingdom).

NRPB (2001). National Radiological Protection Board. *Guidance Notes for Dental Practitioners on the Safe Use of X-ray Equipment* (National Radiation Protection Board, Chilton, United Kingdom).

OSHA (1994a). Occupational Safety and Health Administration. "Hazard communication: Final rule," 59 FR 6126 (U.S. Government Printing Office, Washington).

OSHA (1994b). Occupational Safety and Health Administration. "Personal protective equipment for general industry: final rule," 59 FR 16360 (U.S. Government Printing Office, Washington).

OSHA (2001). Occupational Safety and Health Administration. "Occupational exposure to bloodborne pathogens: Needle sticks and other sharps injuries: Final rule," 66 FR 5317 (U.S. Government Printing Office, Washington).

PIERCE, D.A. and PRESTON, D.L. (2000). "Radiation-related cancer risks at low doses among atomic bomb survivors," Radiat. Res. **154**(2), 178–186.

PLATIN, E., JANHOM, A. and TYNDALL, D. (1998). "A quantitative analysis of dental radiography quality assurance practices among North Carolina dentists," Oral Surg. Oral Med. Oral Pathol. Oral Radiol. Endod. **86**(1), 115–120.

PRESTON, D.L., RON, E., YONEHARA, S., KOBUKE, T., FUJII, H., KISHIKAWA, M., TOKUNGA, M., TOKUOKA, S. and MABUCHI, K. (2002). "Tumors of the nervous system and pituitary gland associated with atomic bomb radiation exposure," J. Natl. Cancer Inst. **94**, 1555–1563.

PRESTON, D.L., SHIMIZU, Y., PIERCE, D.A., SUYAMA, A. and MABUCHI, K. (2003). "Studies of mortality of atomic bomb survivors.

Report 13: Solid cancer and noncancer disease mortality: 1950-1997," Radiat. Res. **160**(4), 381–407.

PRESTON-MARTIN, S., THOMAS, D.C., WHITE, S.C. and COHEN, D. (1988). "Prior exposure to medical and dental x-rays related to tumors of the parotid gland," J. Natl. Cancer Inst. **80**(12), 943–949.

PRESTON-MARTIN, S., MACK, W. and HENDERSON, B.E. (1989). "Risk factors for gliomas and meningiomas in males in Los Angeles County," Cancer Res. **49**(21), 6137–6143.

PRICE, C. (1995). "Sensitometric evaluation of a new E-speed dental radiographic film," Dentomaxillofac. Radiol. **24**(1), 30–36.

PUSKIN, J.S. (2003). "Smoking as a cofounder in ecologic correlations of cancer mortality rates with average county radon levels," Health Phys. **84**, 526–532.

REID, J.A. and MACDONALD, J.C. (1984). "Use and workload factors in dental radiation-protection design," Oral Surg. Oral Med. Oral Pathol. **57**(2), 219–224.

REID, J.A., MACDONALD, J.C., DEKKER, T.A. and KUPPERS, B.U. (1993). "Radiation exposures around a panoramic dental x-ray unit," Oral Surg. Oral Med. Oral Pathol. **75**(6), 780–782.

RON, E. and MODAN, B. (1984). "Thyroid and other neoplasms following childhood scalp irradiation," pages 139 to 152 in *Radiation Carcinogenesis: Epidemiology and Biological Significance*, Boice, J.D., Jr. and Fraumeni, J.F., Jr., Eds. (Raven Press, New York).

RON, E., PRESTON, D.L., MABUCHI, K., THOMPSON, D.E. and SODA, M. (1994). "Cancer incidence in atomic bomb survivors. Part IV: Comparison of cancer incidence and mortality," Radiat. Res. **137**(2), S98–S112.

RON, E., LUBIN, J.H., SHORE, R.E., MABUCHI, K., MODAN, B., POTTERN, L.M., SCHNEIDER, A.B., TUCKER, M.A. and BOICE, J.D., JR. (1995). "Thyroid cancer after exposure to external radiation: A pooled analysis of seven studies," Radiat. Res. **141**(3), 259–277.

RON, E., PRESTON, D.L., KISHIKAWA, M., KOBUKE, T., ISEKI, M., TOKUOKA, S., TOKUNAGA, M., and MABUCHI, K. (1998). "Skin tumor risk among atomic-bomb survivors in Japan," Cancer Causes Control **9**(4), 393–401.

ROWLAND, R.E. and LUCAS, H.F. (1984). "Radium dial workers," pages 231 to 240 in *Radiation Carcinogenesis: Epidemiology and Biological Significance*, Boice, J.D., Jr. and Fraumeni, J.F., Jr., Eds. (Raven Press, New York).

RUBIN, P. and CASARETT, G.W. (1968). *Clinical Radiation Pathology* (W.B. Saunders, Philadelphia).

RUMBERG, H., HOLLENDER, L. and ODA, D. (1996). "Assessing the quality of radiographs accompanying biopsy specimens," J. Am. Dent. Assoc. **127**(3), 363–368.

SANDERINK, G.C., HUISKENS, R., VAN DER STELT, P.F., WELANDER, U.S. and STHEEMAN, S.E. (1994). "Image quality of direct digital intraoral x-ray sensors in assessing root canal length.

The RadioVisioGraphy, Visualix/VIXA, Sens-A-Ray, and Flash Dent systems compared with Ektaspeed films," Oral Surg. Oral Med. Oral Pathol. **78**(1), 125–132.

SHEARER, A.C., HORNER, K. and WILSON, N.H. (1990). "Radiovisiography for imaging root canals: An *in vitro* comparison with conventional radiography," Quintessence Int. **21**(10), 789–794.

SHIMIZU, Y., KATO, H. and SCHULL, W.J. (1990). "Studies of the mortality of A-bomb survivors. 9. Mortality, 1950-1985: Part 2. Cancer mortality based on the recently revised doses (DS86)," Radiat. Res. **121**(2), 120–141.

SHIMIZU, Y., PIERCE, D.A., PRESTON, D.L. and MABUCHI, K. (1999). "Studies of the mortality of atomic bomb survivors. Report 12, Part II. Noncancer mortality: 1950-1990," Radiat. Res. **152**(4), 374–389.

SHORE, R.E., ALBERT, R.E. and PASTERNACK, B.S. (1976). "Follow-up study of patients treated by x-ray epilation for tinea capitis: Resurvey of post-treatment illness and mortality experience," Arch. Environ. Health **31**(1), 21–28.

SIMPKIN, D.J. (1995). "Transmission data for shielding diagnostic x-ray facilities," Health Phys. **68**(5), 704–709.

SIMPKIN, D.J. and DIXON, R.L. (1998). "Secondary shielding barriers for diagnostic x-ray facilities: Scatter and leakage revisited," Health Phys. **74**(3), 350–365.

SVANAES, D.B., MOYSTAD, A., RISNES, S., LARHEIM, T.A. and GRONDAHL, H.G. (1996). "Intraoral storage phosphor radiography for approximal caries detection and effect of image magnification: Comparison with conventional radiography," Oral Surg. Oral Med. Oral Pathol. Oral Radiol. Endod. **82**(1), 94–100.

SVENSON, B. and PETERSSON, A. (1995). "Questionnaire survey on the use of dental x-ray film and equipment among general practitioners in the Swedish Public Dental Health Service," Acta Odontol. Scand. **53**(4), 230–235.

SVENSON, B., SODERFELDT, B. and GRONDAHL, H.G. (1996). "Attitudes of Swedish dentists to the choice of dental x-ray film and collimator for oral radiology," Dentomaxillofac. Radiol. **25**(3), 157–161.

SVENSON, B., WELANDER, U., SHI, X.Q., STAMATAKIS, H. and TRONJE, G. (1997a). "A sensitometric comparison of four dental x-ray films and their diagnostic accuracy," Dentomaxillofac. Radiol. **26**(4), 230–235.

SVENSON, B., SODERFELDT, B. and GRONDAHL, H. (1997b). "Knowledge of radiology among Swedish dentists," Dentomaxillofac. Radiol. **26**(4), 219–224.

SVENSON, B., GRONDAHL, H.G., and SODERFELDT, B. (1998). "A logistic regression model for analyzing the relation between dentists attitudes, behavior, and knowledge in oral radiology," Acta. Odontol. Scand. **56**(4), 215–219.

TAKEICHI, N., DOHI, K., YAMAMOTO, H., ITO, H., MABUCHI, K., YAMAMOTO, T., SHIMAOKA, K. and YOKORO, K. (1991). "Parathyroid tumors in atomic bomb survivors in Hiroshima: Epidemiological study from registered cases at Hiroshima Prefecture Tumor Tissue Registry, 1974-1987," Jpn. J. Cancer Res. **82**(8), 875–878.

TAMBURUS, J.R. and LAVRADOR, M.A. (1997). "Radiographic contrast. A comparative study of three dental x-ray films," Dentomaxillofac. Radiol. **26**(4), 201–205.

THOMPSON, D.E., MABUCHI, K., RON, E., SODA, M., TOKUNAGA, M., OCHIKUBO, S., SUGIMOTO, S., IKEDA, T., TERASAKI, M. and IZUMI, S. et al. (1994). "Cancer incidence in atomic bomb survivors. Part II: Solid tumors, 1958-1987," Radiat. Res. **137**, S17–S67.

THUNTHY, K.H. (2000) "Clinical trial of Kodak™ F-speed film finds contrast, resolution equal to D-speed," Contemp. Esthetics Restorat. Pract. **4**, 38–39.

THUNTHY, K.H. and WEINBERG, R. (1982). "Sensitometric comparison of dental films of groups D and E," Oral Surg. Oral Med. Oral Pathol. **54**(2), 250–252.

THUNTHY, K.H. and WEINBERG, R. (1986). "Sensitometic and image analysis of T-grain film," Oral Surg. Oral Med. Oral Pathol. **62**(2), 218–220.

TJELMELAND, E.M., MOORE, W.S., HERMESCH, C.B. and BUIKEMA, D.J. (1998). "A perceptibility curve comparison of Ultra-Speed and Ektaspeed Plus films," Oral Surg. Oral Med. Oral Pathol. Oral Radiol. Endod. **85**(4), 485–488.

TSANG, A., SWEET, D. and WOOD, R.E. (1999). "Potential for fraudulent use of digital radiography," J. Am. Dent. Assoc. **130**(9), 1325–1329.

UNDERHILL, T.E., CHILVARQUER, I., KIMURA, K., LANGLAIS, R.P., MCDAVID, W.D., PREECE, J.W. and BARNWELL, G. (1988). "Radiobiologic risk estimation from dental radiology. Part I. Absorbed doses to critical organs," Oral Surg. Oral Med. Oral Pathol. **66**(1), 111–120.

UNSCEAR (1993). United Nations Scientific Committee on the Effects of Atomic Radiation. *Sources and Effects of Ionizing Radiation, UNSCEAR 1993 Report to the General Assembly, with Scientific Annexes*, Publication E.94.IX.2 (United Nations, New York).

UNSCEAR (1994). United Nations Scientific Committee on the Effects of Atomic Radiation. *Sources and Effects of Ionizing Radiation, UNSCEAR 1994 Report to the General Assembly, with Scientific Annexes* (United Nations, New York).

UNSCEAR (2000). United Nations Scientific Committee on the Effects of Atomic Radiation. *Sources and Effects of Ionizing Radiation. Volume I, Sources, UNSCEAR 2000 Report to the General Assembly, with References*, Publication E.00.IX.3 (United Nations, New York).

UNSCEAR (2001). United Nations Scientific Committee on the Effects of Atomic Radiation. *Hereditary Effects of Radiation. UNSCEAR 2001 Report to the General Assembly, with Scientific Annexes*, Publication E.01.IX.2 (United Nations, New York).

VALACHOVIC, R.W., REISKIN, A.B. and KIRCHHOF, S.T. (1981). "A quality assurance program in dental radiology," Pediatr. Dent. **3**(1), 26–32.

VAN AKEN, J. and VAN DER LINDEN, L.W. (1966). "The integral absorbed dose in conventional and panoramic complete-mouth examinations," Oral Surg. Oral Med. Oral Pathol. **22**(5), 603–616.

VAN PELT, W.R. (2003). "Epidemiological associations among lung cancer, radon exposure and elevation above sea level—a reassessment of Cohen's county level radon study," Health Phys. **85**(4), 397–403.

WEINBERG, H.S., KOROL, A.B., KIRZHNER, V.M., AVIVI, A., FAHIMA, T., NEVO, E., SHAPIRO, S., RENNERT, G., PIATAK, O., STEPANOVA, E.I. and SKVARSKAJA, E. (2001). "Very high mutation rate in offspring of Chernobyl accident liquidators," Proc. R. Soc. London B. Biol. Sci. **268**, 1001–1005.

WENZEL, A. and GRONDAHL, H.G. (1995). "Direct digital radiography in the dental office," Int. Dent. J. **45**(1), 27–34.

WHITE, S.C. (1992). "1992 assessment of radiation risk from dental radiography," Dentomaxillofac. Radiol. **21**(3), 118–126.

WHITE, S.C. and PHARAOH, M.J. (2004). *Oral Radiology: Principles and Interpretation*, 5th ed. (Mosby, St. Louis, Missouri).

WILLIAMS, J.R. and MONTGOMERY, A. (2000). "Measurement of dose in panoramic dental radiology," Br. J. Radiol. **73**, 1002–1006.

WUEHRMANN, A.H. (1970). "Radiation hygiene and its practice in dentistry as related to film viewing procedures and radiographic interpretation. Council on Dental Materials and Devices," J. Am. Dent. Assoc. **80**(2), 346–356.

The NCRP

The National Council on Radiation Protection and Measurements is a nonprofit corporation chartered by Congress in 1964 to:

1. Collect, analyze, develop and disseminate in the public interest information and recommendations about (a) protection against radiation and (b) radiation measurements, quantities and units, particularly those concerned with radiation protection.
2. Provide a means by which organizations concerned with the scientific and related aspects of radiation protection and of radiation quantities, units and measurements may cooperate for effective utilization of their combined resources, and to stimulate the work of such organizations.
3. Develop basic concepts about radiation quantities, units and measurements, about the application of these concepts, and about radiation protection.
4. Cooperate with the International Commission on Radiological Protection, the International Commission on Radiation Units and Measurements, and other national and international organizations, governmental and private, concerned with radiation quantities, units and measurements and with radiation protection.

The Council is the successor to the unincorporated association of scientists known as the National Committee on Radiation Protection and Measurements and was formed to carry on the work begun by the Committee in 1929.

The participants in the Council's work are the Council members and members of scientific and administrative committees. Council members are selected solely on the basis of their scientific expertise and serve as individuals, not as representatives of any particular organization. The scientific committees, composed of experts having detailed knowledge and competence in the particular area of the committee's interest, draft proposed recommendations. These are then submitted to the full membership of the Council for careful review and approval before being published.

The following comprise the current officers and membership of the Council:

Officers

President	Thomas S. Tenforde
Senior Vice President	Kenneth R. Kase
Secretary and Treasurer	William M. Beckner
Assistant Secretary	Michael F. McBride

Members

John F. Ahearne
Larry E. Anderson
Benjamin R. Archer
Mary M. Austin-Seymour
Harold L. Beck
Eleanor A. Blakely
William F. Blakely
John D. Boice, Jr.
Thomas B. Borak
Andre Bouville
Leslie A. Braby
David Brenner
Antone L. Brooks
Jerrold T. Bushberg
John F. Cardella
Stephanie K. Carlson
S.Y. Chen
Chung-Kwang Chou
Kelly L. Classic
Mary E. Clark
James E. Cleaver
J. Donald Cossairt
Allen G. Croff
Francis A. Cucinotta
Carter Denniston
Paul M. DeLuca
John F. Dicello, Jr.
Sarah S. Donaldson
William P. Dornsife
Stephen A. Feig
H. Keith Florig
Kenneth R. Foster
John R. Frazier
Thomas F. Gesell
Ethel S. Gilbert
Joel E. Gray
Andrew J. Grosovsky
Raymond A. Guilmette
Roger W. Harms
John W. Hirshfeld, Jr.
David G. Hoel
F. Owen Hoffman
Roger W. Howell
Kenneth R. Kase
Ann R. Kennedy
David C. Kocher
Ritsuko Komaki
Amy Kronenberg
Charles E. Land
Susan M. Langhorst
Richard W. Leggett
Howard L. Liber
James C. Lin
Jill A. Lipoti
John B. Little
Jay H. Lubin
C. Douglas Maynard
Claire M. Mays
Cynthia H. McCollough
Barbara J. McNeil
Fred A. Mettler, Jr.
Charles W. Miller
Jack Miller
Kenneth L. Miller
William F. Morgan
John E. Moulder
David S. Myers
Bruce A. Napier
Carl J. Paperiello
Ronald C. Petersen
R. Julian Preston
Jerome S. Puskin
Allan C.B. Richardson
Henry D. Royal
Marvin Rosenstein
Lawrence N. Rothenberg
Michael T. Ryan
Jonathan M. Samet
Stephen M. Seltzer
Roy E. Shore
Edward A. Sickles
David H. Sliney
Paul Slovic
Daniel J. Strom
Thomas S. Tenforde
Lawrence W. Townsend
Lois B. Travis
Robert L. Ullrich
Richard J. Vetter
Daniel E. Wartenberg
David A. Weber
F. Ward Whicker
Chris G. Whipple
J. Frank Wilson
Susan D. Wiltshire
Gayle E. Woloschak
Marco A. Zaider
Pasquale D. Zanzonico
Marvin C. Ziskin

Honorary Members

Lauriston S. Taylor, *Honorary President*
Warren K. Sinclair, *President Emeritus;* Charles B. Meinhold, *President Emeritus*
S. James Adelstein, *Honorary Vice President*
W. Roger Ney, *Executive Director Emeritus*

Seymour Abrahamson
Edward L. Alpen
Lynn R. Anspaugh
John A. Auxier
William J. Bair
Bruce B. Boecker
Victor P. Bond
Robert L. Brent
Reynold F. Brown
Melvin C. Carter
Randall S. Caswell
Frederick P. Cowan
James F. Crow
Gerald D. Dodd
Patricia W. Durbin
Keith F. Eckerman
Thomas S. Ely
Richard F. Foster
R.J. Michael Fry
Robert O. Gorson
Arthur W. Guy
Eric J. Hall
Naomi H. Harley
William R. Hendee
Donald G. Jacobs
Bernd Kahn
Roger O. McClellan
Dade W. Moeller
A. Alan Moghissi
Wesley L. Nyborg
John W. Poston, Sr.
Andrew K. Poznanski
Chester R. Richmond
Genevieve S. Roessler
Eugene L. Saenger
William J. Schull
J. Newell Stannard
John B. Storer
John E. Till
Arthur C. Upton
Edward W. Webster

Lauriston S. Taylor Lecturers

Charles B. Meinhold (2003) *The Evolution of Radiation Protection: From Erythema to Genetic Risks to Risks of Cancer to ?*

R. Julian Preston (2002) *Developing Mechanistic Data for Incorporation into Cancer Risk Assessment: Old Problems and New Approaches*

Wesley L. Nyborg (2001) *Assuring the Safety of Medical Diagnostic Ultrasound*

S. James Adelstein (2000) *Administered Radioactivity: Unde Venimus Quoque Imus*

Naomi H. Harley (1999) *Back to Background*

Eric J. Hall (1998) *From Chimney Sweeps to Astronauts: Cancer Risks in the Workplace*

William J. Bair (1997) *Radionuclides in the Body: Meeting the Challenge!*

Seymour Abrahamson (1996) *70 Years of Radiation Genetics: Fruit Flies, Mice and Humans*

Albrecht Kellerer (1995) *Certainty and Uncertainty in Radiation Protection*

R.J. Michael Fry (1994) *Mice, Myths and Men*

Warren K. Sinclair (1993) *Science, Radiation Protection and the NCRP*

Edward W. Webster (1992) *Dose and Risk in Diagnostic Radiology: How Big? How Little?*

Victor P. Bond (1991) *When is a Dose Not a Dose?*

J. Newell Stannard (1990) *Radiation Protection and the Internal Emitter Saga*

Arthur C. Upton (1989) *Radiobiology and Radiation Protection: The Past Century and Prospects for the Future*

Bo Lindell (1988) *How Safe is Safe Enough?*

Seymour Jablon (1987) *How to be Quantitative about Radiation Risk Estimates*

Herman P. Schwan (1986) *Biological Effects of Non-ionizing Radiations: Cellular Properties and Interactions*

John H. Harley (1985) *Truth (and Beauty) in Radiation Measurement*

Harald H. Rossi (1984) *Limitation and Assessment in Radiation Protection*

Merril Eisenbud (1983) *The Human Environment—Past, Present and Future*

Eugene L. Saenger (1982) *Ethics, Trade-Offs and Medical Radiation*

James F. Crow (1981) *How Well Can We Assess Genetic Risk? Not Very*

Harold O. Wyckoff (1980) *From "Quantity of Radiation" and "Dose" to "Exposure" and "Absorbed Dose"—An Historical Review*

Hymer L. Friedell (1979) *Radiation Protection—Concepts and Trade Offs*

Sir Edward Pochin (1978) *Why be Quantitative about Radiation Risk Estimates?*

Herbert M. Parker (1977) *The Squares of the Natural Numbers in Radiation Protection*

Currently, the following committees are actively engaged in formulating recommendations:

SC 1 Basic Criteria, Epidemiology, Radiobiology and Risk
 SC 1-4 Extrapolation of Risks from Non-human Experimental Systems to Man
 SC 1-7 Information Needed to Make Radiation Protection Recommendations for Travel Beyond Low-Earth Orbit
 SC 1-8 Risk to Thyroid from Ionizing Radiation
 SC 1-10 Review of Cohen's Radon Research Methods
SC 9 Structural Shielding Design and Evaluation for Medical Use of X Rays and Gamma Rays of Energies Up to 10 MeV
SC 46 Operational Radiation Safety
 SC 46-13 Design of Facilities for Medical Radiation Therapy
 SC 46-16 Radiation Protection in Veterinary Medicine
 SC 46-17 Radiation Protection in Educational Institutions
 SC 57-15 Uranium Risk
 SC 57-17 Radionuclide Dosimetry Models for Wounds
SC 64 Environmental Issues
 SC 64-22 Design of Effective Effluent and Environmental Monitoring Programs
 SC 64-23 Cesium in the Environment
SC 72 Radiation Protection in Mammography
SC 85 Risk of Lung Cancer from Radon
SC 87 Radioactive and Mixed Waste
 SC 87-3 Performance Assessment of Near Surface Radioactive Waste Facilities
 SC 87-5 Risk Management Analysis for Decommissioned Sites
SC 89 Nonionizing Radiation
 SC 89-3 Biological Effects of Extremely Low-Frequency Electric and Magnetic Fields
 SC 89-5 Biological Effects of Radiofrequency Electromagnetic Fields
SC 91 Radiation Protection in Medicine
 SC 91-1 Precautions in the Management of Patients Who Have Received Therapeutic Amounts of Radionuclides
SC 92 Public Policy and Risk Communication
SC 93 Radiation Measurement and Dosimetry

In recognition of its responsibility to facilitate and stimulate cooperation among organizations concerned with the scientific and related aspects of radiation protection and measurement, the Council has created a category of NCRP Collaborating Organizations. Organizations or groups of organizations that are national or international in scope and are concerned with scientific problems involving radiation quantities, units, measurements and effects, or radiation protection may be admitted to collaborating status by the Council. Collaborating Organizations provide a means by which the NCRP can gain input into its activities from a wider segment of society. At the same time, the relationships with the Collaborating Organizations facilitate wider dissemination of information about the Council's activities, interests and concerns. Collaborating Organizations have the opportunity to comment on draft reports (at the time that these are submitted to the members of the Council). This is intended to capitalize on the fact that Collaborating Organizations are in an excellent position to both contribute to the identification of what needs to be treated in NCRP reports and to identify problems that might result from proposed recommendations. The present Collaborating Organizations with which the NCRP maintains liaison are as follows:

Agency for Toxic Substances and Disease Registry
American Academy of Dermatology
American Academy of Environmental Engineers
American Academy of Health Physics
American Association of Physicists in Medicine
American College of Medical Physics
American College of Nuclear Physicians
American College of Occupational and Environmental Medicine
American College of Radiology
American Dental Association
American Industrial Hygiene Association
American Institute of Ultrasound in Medicine
American Insurance Services Group
American Medical Association
American Nuclear Society
American Pharmaceutical Association
American Podiatric Medical Association
American Public Health Association
American Radium Society
American Roentgen Ray Society
American Society for Therapeutic Radiology and Oncology
American Society of Emergency Radiology
American Society of Health-System Pharmacists
American Society of Radiologic Technologists
Association of Educators in Radiological Sciences, Inc.
Association of University Radiologists
Bioelectromagnetics Society
Campus Radiation Safety Officers
College of American Pathologists
Conference of Radiation Control Program Directors, Inc.
Council on Radionuclides and Radiopharmaceuticals
Defense Threat Reduction Agency
Electric Power Research Institute
Federal Communications Commission
Federal Emergency Management Agency
Genetics Society of America

Health Physics Society
Institute of Electrical and Electronics Engineers, Inc.
Institute of Nuclear Power Operations
International Brotherhood of Electrical Workers
National Aeronautics and Space Administration
National Association of Environmental Professionals
National Electrical Manufacturers Association
National Institute for Occupational Safety and Health
National Institute of Standards and Technology
Nuclear Energy Institute
Office of Science and Technology Policy
Paper, Allied-Industrial, Chemical and Energy Workers International Union
Product Stewardship Institute
Radiation Research Society
Radiological Society of North America
Society for Risk Analysis
Society of Chairmen of Academic Radiology Departments
Society of Nuclear Medicine
Society of Radiologists in Ultrasound
Society of Skeletal Radiology
U.S. Air Force
U.S. Army
U.S. Coast Guard
U.S. Department of Energy
U.S. Department of Housing and Urban Development
U.S. Department of Labor
U.S. Department of Transportation
U.S. Environmental Protection Agency
U.S. Navy
U.S. Nuclear Regulatory Commission
U.S. Public Health Service
Utility Workers Union of America

The NCRP has found its relationships with these organizations to be extremely valuable to continued progress in its program.

Another aspect of the cooperative efforts of the NCRP relates to the Special Liaison relationships established with various governmental organizations that have an interest in radiation protection and measurements. This liaison relationship provides: (1) an opportunity for participating organizations to designate an individual to provide liaison between the organization and the NCRP; (2) that the individual designated will receive copies of draft NCRP reports (at the time that these are submitted to the members of the Council) with an invitation to comment, but not vote; and (3) that new NCRP efforts might be discussed with liaison individuals as appropriate, so that they might have an opportunity to make suggestions on new studies and related matters. The following organizations participate in the Special Liaison Program:

Australian Radiation Laboratory
Bundesamt für Strahlenschutz (Germany)
Canadian Nuclear Safety Commission
Central Laboratory for Radiological Protection (Poland)
China Institute for Radiation Protection
Commisariat à l'Energie Atomique
Commonwealth Scientific Instrumentation Research Organization (Australia)
European Commission
Health Council of the Netherlands
International Commission on Non-ionizing Radiation Protection
Japan Radiation Council
Korea Institute of Nuclear Safety
National Radiological Protection Board (United Kingdom)
Russian Scientific Commission on Radiation Protection
South African Forum for Radiation Protection
World Association of Nuclear Operations

The NCRP values highly the participation of these organizations in the Special Liaison Program.

The Council also benefits significantly from the relationships established pursuant to the Corporate Sponsor's Program. The program facilitates the interchange of information and ideas and corporate sponsors provide valuable fiscal support for the Council's program. This developing program currently includes the following Corporate Sponsors:

3M Corporate Health Physics
Amersham Health
Duke Energy Corporation
ICN Biomedicals, Inc.
Landauer, Inc.
Nuclear Energy Institute
Philips Medical Systems
Southern California Edison

The Council's activities are made possible by the voluntary contribution of time and effort by its members and participants and the generous support of the following organizations:

3M Health Physics Services
Agfa Corporation
Alfred P. Sloan Foundation
Alliance of American Insurers
American Academy of Dermatology
American Academy of Health Physics
American Academy of Oral and Maxillofacial Radiology

American Association of Physicists in Medicine
American Cancer Society
American College of Medical Physics
American College of Nuclear Physicians
American College of Occupational and Environmental Medicine
American College of Radiology
American College of Radiology Foundation
American Dental Association
American Healthcare Radiology Administrators
American Industrial Hygiene Association
American Insurance Services Group
American Medical Association
American Nuclear Society
American Osteopathic College of Radiology
American Podiatric Medical Association
American Public Health Association
American Radium Society
American Roentgen Ray Society
American Society of Radiologic Technologists
American Society for Therapeutic Radiology and Oncology
American Veterinary Medical Association
American Veterinary Radiology Society
Association of Educators in Radiological Sciences, Inc.
Association of University Radiologists
Battelle Memorial Institute
Canberra Industries, Inc.
Chem Nuclear Systems
Center for Devices and Radiological Health
College of American Pathologists
Committee on Interagency Radiation Research
and Policy Coordination
Commonwealth Edison
Commonwealth of Pennsylvania
Consolidated Edison
Consumers Power Company
Council on Radionuclides and Radiopharmaceuticals
Defense Nuclear Agency
Eastman Kodak Company
Edison Electric Institute
Edward Mallinckrodt, Jr. Foundation
EG&G Idaho, Inc.
Electric Power Research Institute
Electromagnetic Energy Association
Federal Emergency Management Agency
Florida Institute of Phosphate Research
Florida Power Corporation
Fuji Medical Systems, U.S.A., Inc.

Genetics Society of America
Health Effects Research Foundation (Japan)
Health Physics Society
Institute of Nuclear Power Operations
James Picker Foundation
Martin Marietta Corporation
Motorola Foundation
National Aeronautics and Space Administration
National Association of Photographic Manufacturers
National Cancer Institute
National Electrical Manufacturers Association
National Institute of Standards and Technology
New York Power Authority
Picker International
Public Service Electric and Gas Company
Radiation Research Society
Radiological Society of North America
Richard Lounsbery Foundation
Sandia National Laboratory
Siemens Medical Systems, Inc.
Society of Nuclear Medicine
Society of Pediatric Radiology
U.S. Department of Energy
U.S. Department of Labor
U.S. Environmental Protection Agency
U.S. Navy
U.S. Nuclear Regulatory Commission
Victoreen, Inc.
Westinghouse Electric Corporation

Initial funds for publication of NCRP reports were provided by a grant from the James Picker Foundation.

The NCRP seeks to promulgate information and recommendations based on leading scientific judgment on matters of radiation protection and measurement and to foster cooperation among organizations concerned with these matters. These efforts are intended to serve the public interest and the Council welcomes comments and suggestions on its reports or activities from those interested in its work.

NCRP Publications

Information on NCRP publications may be obtained from the NCRP website (http://www.ncrp.com) or by telephone (800-229-2652, ext. 25) and fax (301-907-8768). The address is:

NCRP Publications
7910 Woodmont Avenue
Suite 400
Bethesda, MD 20814-3095

Abstracts of NCRP reports published since 1980, abstracts of all NCRP commentaries, and the text of all NCRP statements are available at the NCRP website. Currently available publications are listed below.

NCRP Reports

No.	Title
8	*Control and Removal of Radioactive Contamination in Laboratories* (1951)
22	*Maximum Permissible Body Burdens and Maximum Permissible Concentrations of Radionuclides in Air and in Water for Occupational Exposure* (1959) [includes Addendum 1 issued in August 1963]
25	*Measurement of Absorbed Dose of Neutrons, and of Mixtures of Neutrons and Gamma Rays* (1961)
27	*Stopping Powers for Use with Cavity Chambers* (1961)
30	*Safe Handling of Radioactive Materials* (1964)
32	*Radiation Protection in Educational Institutions* (1966)
35	*Dental X-Ray Protection* (1970)
36	*Radiation Protection in Veterinary Medicine* (1970)
37	*Precautions in the Management of Patients Who Have Received Therapeutic Amounts of Radionuclides* (1970)
38	*Protection Against Neutron Radiation* (1971)
40	*Protection Against Radiation from Brachytherapy Sources* (1972)
41	*Specification of Gamma-Ray Brachytherapy Sources* (1974)

42 *Radiological Factors Affecting Decision-Making in a Nuclear Attack* (1974)
44 *Krypton-85 in the Atmosphere—Accumulation, Biological Significance, and Control Technology* (1975)
46 *Alpha-Emitting Particles in Lungs* (1975)
47 *Tritium Measurement Techniques* (1976)
49 *Structural Shielding Design and Evaluation for Medical Use of X Rays and Gamma Rays of Energies Up to 10 MeV* (1976)
50 *Environmental Radiation Measurements* (1976)
52 *Cesium-137 from the Environment to Man: Metabolism and Dose* (1977)
54 *Medical Radiation Exposure of Pregnant and Potentially Pregnant Women* (1977)
55 *Protection of the Thyroid Gland in the Event of Releases of Radioiodine* (1977)
57 *Instrumentation and Monitoring Methods for Radiation Protection* (1978)
58 *A Handbook of Radioactivity Measurements Procedures*, 2nd ed. (1985)
60 *Physical, Chemical, and Biological Properties of Radiocerium Relevant to Radiation Protection Guidelines* (1978)
61 *Radiation Safety Training Criteria for Industrial Radiography* (1978)
62 *Tritium in the Environment* (1979)
63 *Tritium and Other Radionuclide Labeled Organic Compounds Incorporated in Genetic Material* (1979)
64 *Influence of Dose and Its Distribution in Time on Dose-Response Relationships for Low-LET Radiations* (1980)
65 *Management of Persons Accidentally Contaminated with Radionuclides* (1980)
67 *Radiofrequency Electromagnetic Fields—Properties, Quantities and Units, Biophysical Interaction, and Measurements* (1981)
68 *Radiation Protection in Pediatric Radiology* (1981)
69 *Dosimetry of X-Ray and Gamma-Ray Beams for Radiation Therapy in the Energy Range 10 keV to 50 MeV* (1981)
70 *Nuclear Medicine—Factors Influencing the Choice and Use of Radionuclides in Diagnosis and Therapy* (1982)
72 *Radiation Protection and Measurement for Low-Voltage Neutron Generators* (1983)
73 *Protection in Nuclear Medicine and Ultrasound Diagnostic Procedures in Children* (1983)
74 *Biological Effects of Ultrasound: Mechanisms and Clinical Implications* (1983)
75 *Iodine-129: Evaluation of Releases from Nuclear Power Generation* (1983)
77 *Exposures from the Uranium Series with Emphasis on Radon and Its Daughters* (1984)

78 *Evaluation of Occupational and Environmental Exposures to Radon and Radon Daughters in the United States* (1984)
79 *Neutron Contamination from Medical Electron Accelerators* (1984)
80 *Induction of Thyroid Cancer by Ionizing Radiation* (1985)
81 *Carbon-14 in the Environment* (1985)
82 *SI Units in Radiation Protection and Measurements* (1985)
83 *The Experimental Basis for Absorbed-Dose Calculations in Medical Uses of Radionuclides* (1985)
84 *General Concepts for the Dosimetry of Internally Deposited Radionuclides* (1985)
85 *Mammography—A User's Guide* (1986)
86 *Biological Effects and Exposure Criteria for Radiofrequency Electromagnetic Fields* (1986)
87 *Use of Bioassay Procedures for Assessment of Internal Radionuclide Deposition* (1987)
88 *Radiation Alarms and Access Control Systems* (1986)
89 *Genetic Effects from Internally Deposited Radionuclides* (1987)
90 *Neptunium: Radiation Protection Guidelines* (1988)
92 *Public Radiation Exposure from Nuclear Power Generation in the United States* (1987)
93 *Ionizing Radiation Exposure of the Population of the United States* (1987)
94 *Exposure of the Population in the United States and Canada from Natural Background Radiation* (1987)
95 *Radiation Exposure of the U.S. Population from Consumer Products and Miscellaneous Sources* (1987)
96 *Comparative Carcinogenicity of Ionizing Radiation and Chemicals* (1989)
97 *Measurement of Radon and Radon Daughters in Air* (1988)
99 *Quality Assurance for Diagnostic Imaging* (1988)
100 *Exposure of the U.S. Population from Diagnostic Medical Radiation* (1989)
101 *Exposure of the U.S. Population from Occupational Radiation* (1989)
102 *Medical X-Ray, Electron Beam and Gamma-Ray Protection for Energies Up to 50 MeV (Equipment Design, Performance and Use)* (1989)
103 *Control of Radon in Houses* (1989)
104 *The Relative Biological Effectiveness of Radiations of Different Quality* (1990)
105 *Radiation Protection for Medical and Allied Health Personnel* (1989)
106 *Limit for Exposure to "Hot Particles" on the Skin* (1989)
107 *Implementation of the Principle of As Low As Reasonably Achievable (ALARA) for Medical and Dental Personnel* (1990)

108 *Conceptual Basis for Calculations of Absorbed-Dose Distributions* (1991)
109 *Effects of Ionizing Radiation on Aquatic Organisms* (1991)
110 *Some Aspects of Strontium Radiobiology* (1991)
111 *Developing Radiation Emergency Plans for Academic, Medical or Industrial Facilities* (1991)
112 *Calibration of Survey Instruments Used in Radiation Protection for the Assessment of Ionizing Radiation Fields and Radioactive Surface Contamination* (1991)
113 *Exposure Criteria for Medical Diagnostic Ultrasound: I. Criteria Based on Thermal Mechanisms* (1992)
114 *Maintaining Radiation Protection Records* (1992)
115 *Risk Estimates for Radiation Protection* (1993)
116 *Limitation of Exposure to Ionizing Radiation* (1993)
117 *Research Needs for Radiation Protection* (1993)
118 *Radiation Protection in the Mineral Extraction Industry* (1993)
119 *A Practical Guide to the Determination of Human Exposure to Radiofrequency Fields* (1993)
120 *Dose Control at Nuclear Power Plants* (1994)
121 *Principles and Application of Collective Dose in Radiation Protection* (1995)
122 *Use of Personal Monitors to Estimate Effective Dose Equivalent and Effective Dose to Workers for External Exposure to Low-LET Radiation* (1995)
123 *Screening Models for Releases of Radionuclides to Atmosphere, Surface Water, and Ground* (1996)
124 *Sources and Magnitude of Occupational and Public Exposures from Nuclear Medicine Procedures* (1996)
125 *Deposition, Retention and Dosimetry of Inhaled Radioactive Substances* (1997)
126 *Uncertainties in Fatal Cancer Risk Estimates Used in Radiation Protection* (1997)
127 *Operational Radiation Safety Program* (1998)
128 *Radionuclide Exposure of the Embryo/Fetus* (1998)
129 *Recommended Screening Limits for Contaminated Surface Soil and Review of Factors Relevant to Site-Specific Studies* (1999)
130 *Biological Effects and Exposure Limits for "Hot Particles"* (1999)
131 *Scientific Basis for Evaluating the Risks to Populations from Space Applications of Plutonium* (2001)
132 *Radiation Protection Guidance for Activities in Low-Earth Orbit* (2000)
133 *Radiation Protection for Procedures Performed Outside the Radiology Department* (2000)
134 *Operational Radiation Safety Training* (2000)
135 *Liver Cancer Risk from Internally-Deposited Radionuclides* (2001)
136 *Evaluation of the Linear-Nonthreshold Dose-Response Model for Ionizing Radiation* (2001)

137 *Fluence-Based and Microdosimetric Event-Based Methods for Radiation Protection in Space* (2001)
138 *Management of Terrorist Events Involving Radioactive Material* (2001)
139 *Risk-Based Classification of Radioactive and Hazardous Chemical Wastes* (2002)
140 *Exposure Criteria for Medical Diagnostic Ultrasound: II. Criteria Based on all Known Mechanisms* (2002)
141 *Managing Potentially Radioactive Scrap Metal* (2002)
142 *Operational Radiation Safety Program for Astronauts in Low-Earth Orbit: A Basic Framework* (2002)
143 *Management Techniques for Laboratories and Other Small Institutional Generators to Minimize Off-Site Disposal of Low-Level Radioactive Waste* (2003)
144 *Radiation Protection for Particle Accelerator Facilities* (2003)
145 *Radiation Protection in Dentistry* (2003)

Binders for NCRP reports are available. Two sizes make it possible to collect into small binders the "old series" of reports (NCRP Reports Nos. 8–30) and into large binders the more recent publications (NCRP Reports Nos. 32–145). Each binder will accommodate from five to seven reports. The binders carry the identification "NCRP Reports" and come with label holders which permit the user to attach labels showing the reports contained in each binder.

The following bound sets of NCRP reports are also available:

Volume I. NCRP Reports Nos. 8, 22
Volume II. NCRP Reports Nos. 23, 25, 27, 30
Volume III. NCRP Reports Nos. 32, 35, 36, 37
Volume IV. NCRP Reports Nos. 38, 40, 41
Volume V. NCRP Reports Nos. 42, 44, 46
Volume VI. NCRP Reports Nos. 47, 49, 50, 51
Volume VII. NCRP Reports Nos. 52, 53, 54, 55, 57
Volume VIII. NCRP Report No. 58
Volume IX. NCRP Reports Nos. 59, 60, 61, 62, 63
Volume X. NCRP Reports Nos. 64, 65, 66, 67
Volume XI. NCRP Reports Nos. 68, 69, 70, 71, 72
Volume XII. NCRP Reports Nos. 73, 74, 75, 76
Volume XIII. NCRP Reports Nos. 77, 78, 79, 80
Volume XIV. NCRP Reports Nos. 81, 82, 83, 84, 85
Volume XV. NCRP Reports Nos. 86, 87, 88, 89
Volume XVI. NCRP Reports Nos. 90, 91, 92, 93
Volume XVII. NCRP Reports Nos. 94, 95, 96, 97
Volume XVIII. NCRP Reports Nos. 98, 99, 100
Volume XIX. NCRP Reports Nos. 101, 102, 103, 104
Volume XX. NCRP Reports Nos. 105, 106, 107, 108

Volume XXI. NCRP Reports Nos. 109, 110, 111
Volume XXII. NCRP Reports Nos. 112, 113, 114
Volume XXIII. NCRP Reports Nos. 115, 116, 117, 118
Volume XXIV. NCRP Reports Nos. 119, 120, 121, 122
Volume XXV. NCRP Report No. 123I and 123II
Volume XXVI. NCRP Reports Nos. 124, 125, 126, 127
Volume XXVII. NCRP Reports Nos. 128, 129, 130
Volume XXVIII. NCRP Reports Nos. 131, 132, 133
Volume XXIX. NCRP Reports Nos. 134, 135, 136, 137
Volume XXX. NCRP Reports Nos. 138, 139
Volume XXXI. NCRP Report No. 140

(Titles of the individual reports contained in each volume are given previously.)

NCRP Commentaries

No.	Title
1	*Krypton-85 in the Atmosphere—With Specific Reference to the Public Health Significance of the Proposed Controlled Release at Three Mile Island* (1980)
4	*Guidelines for the Release of Waste Water from Nuclear Facilities with Special Reference to the Public Health Significance of the Proposed Release of Treated Waste Waters at Three Mile Island* (1987)
5	*Review of the Publication, Living Without Landfills* (1989)
6	*Radon Exposure of the U.S. Population—Status of the Problem* (1991)
7	*Misadministration of Radioactive Material in Medicine—Scientific Background* (1991)
8	*Uncertainty in NCRP Screening Models Relating to Atmospheric Transport, Deposition and Uptake by Humans* (1993)
9	*Considerations Regarding the Unintended Radiation Exposure of the Embryo, Fetus or Nursing Child* (1994)
10	*Advising the Public about Radiation Emergencies: A Document for Public Comment* (1994)
11	*Dose Limits for Individuals Who Receive Exposure from Radionuclide Therapy Patients* (1995)
12	*Radiation Exposure and High-Altitude Flight* (1995)
13	*An Introduction to Efficacy in Diagnostic Radiology and Nuclear Medicine (Justification of Medical Radiation Exposure)* (1995)
14	*A Guide for Uncertainty Analysis in Dose and Risk Assessments Related to Environmental Contamination* (1996)

15 *Evaluating the Reliability of Biokinetic and Dosimetric Models and Parameters Used to Assess Individual Doses for Risk Assessment Purposes* (1998)
16 *Screening of Humans for Security Purposes Using Ionizing Radiation Scanning Systems* (2003)
17 *Pulsed Fast Neutron Analysis System Used in Security Surveillance* (2003)
18 *Biological Effects of Modulated Radiofrequency Fields* (2003)

Proceedings of the Annual Meeting

No. Title

1 *Perceptions of Risk*, Proceedings of the Fifteenth Annual Meeting held on March 14-15, 1979 (including Taylor Lecture No. 3) (1980)
3 *Critical Issues in Setting Radiation Dose Limits*, Proceedings of the Seventeenth Annual Meeting held on April 8-9, 1981 (including Taylor Lecture No. 5) (1982)
4 *Radiation Protection and New Medical Diagnostic Approaches,* Proceedings of the Eighteenth Annual Meeting held on April 6-7, 1982 (including Taylor Lecture No. 6) (1983)
5 *Environmental Radioactivity,* Proceedings of the Nineteenth Annual Meeting held on April 6-7, 1983 (including Taylor Lecture No. 7) (1983)
6 *Some Issues Important in Developing Basic Radiation Protection Recommendations*, Proceedings of the Twentieth Annual Meeting held on April 4-5, 1984 (including Taylor Lecture No. 8) (1985)
7 *Radioactive Waste*, Proceedings of the Twenty-first Annual Meeting held on April 3-4, 1985 (including Taylor Lecture No. 9)(1986)
8 *Nonionizing Electromagnetic Radiations and Ultrasound,* Proceedings of the Twenty-second Annual Meeting held on April 2-3, 1986 (including Taylor Lecture No. 10) (1988)
9 *New Dosimetry at Hiroshima and Nagasaki and Its Implications for Risk Estimates*, Proceedings of the Twenty-third Annual Meeting held on April 8-9, 1987 (including Taylor Lecture No. 11) (1988)
10 *Radon*, Proceedings of the Twenty-fourth Annual Meeting held on March 30-31, 1988 (including Taylor Lecture No. 12) (1989)
11 *Radiation Protection Today—The NCRP at Sixty Years*, Proceedings of the Twenty-fifth Annual Meeting held on April 5-6, 1989 (including Taylor Lecture No. 13) (1990)
12 *Health and Ecological Implications of Radioactively Contaminated Environments*, Proceedings of the Twenty-sixth

Annual Meeting held on April 4-5, 1990 (including Taylor Lecture No. 14) (1991)

13 *Genes, Cancer and Radiation Protection,* Proceedings of the Twenty-seventh Annual Meeting held on April 3-4, 1991 (including Taylor Lecture No. 15) (1992)

14 *Radiation Protection in Medicine,* Proceedings of the Twenty-eighth Annual Meeting held on April 1-2, 1992 (including Taylor Lecture No. 16) (1993)

15 *Radiation Science and Societal Decision Making,* Proceedings of the Twenty-ninth Annual Meeting held on April 7-8, 1993 (including Taylor Lecture No. 17) (1994)

16 *Extremely-Low-Frequency Electromagnetic Fields: Issues in Biological Effects and Public Health*, Proceedings of the Thirtieth Annual Meeting held on April 6-7, 1994 (not published).

17 *Environmental Dose Reconstruction and Risk Implications,* Proceedings of the Thirty-first Annual Meeting held on April 12-13, 1995 (including Taylor Lecture No. 19) (1996)

18 *Implications of New Data on Radiation Cancer Risk*, Proceedings of the Thirty-second Annual Meeting held on April 3-4, 1996 (including Taylor Lecture No. 20) (1997)

19 *The Effects of Pre- and Postconception Exposure to Radiation*, Proceedings of the Thirty-third Annual Meeting held on April 2-3, 1997, Teratology **59**, 181–317 (1999)

20 *Cosmic Radiation Exposure of Airline Crews, Passengers and Astronauts*, Proceedings of the Thirty-fourth Annual Meeting held on April 1-2, 1998, Health Phys. **79**, 466–613 (2000)

21 *Radiation Protection in Medicine: Contemporary Issues,* Proceedings of the Thirty-fifth Annual Meeting held on April 7-8, 1999 (including Taylor Lecture No. 23) (1999)

22 *Ionizing Radiation Science and Protection in the 21st Century,* Proceedings of the Thirty-sixth Annual Meeting held on April 5-6, 2000, Health Phys. **80**, 317–402 (2001)

23 *Fallout from Atmospheric Nuclear Tests—Impact on Science and Society,* Proceedings of the Thirty-seventh Annual Meeting held on April 4-5, 2001, Health Phys. **82**, 573–748 (2002)

24 *Where the New Biology Meets Epidemiology: Impact on Radiation Risk Estimates*, Proceedings of the Thirty-eighth Annual Meeting held on April 10-11, 2002, Health Phys. **85**, 1–108 (2003).

Lauriston S. Taylor Lectures

No.	Title
1	*The Squares of the Natural Numbers in Radiation Protection by* Herbert M. Parker (1977)
2	*Why be Quantitative about Radiation Risk Estimates?* by Sir Edward Pochin (1978)
3	*Radiation Protection—Concepts and Trade Offs* by Hymer L. Friedell (1979) [available also in *Perceptions of Risk*, see above]
4	*From "Quantity of Radiation" and "Dose" to "Exposure" and "Absorbed Dose"—An Historical Review* by Harold O. Wyckoff (1980)
5	*How Well Can We Assess Genetic Risk? Not Very* by James F. Crow (1981) [available also in *Critical Issues in Setting Radiation Dose Limits*, see above]
6	*Ethics, Trade-offs and Medical Radiation* by Eugene L. Saenger (1982) [available also in *Radiation Protection and New Medical Diagnostic Approaches*, see above]
7	*The Human Environment—Past, Present and Future* by Merril Eisenbud (1983) [available also in *Environmental Radioactivity*, see above]
8	*Limitation and Assessment in Radiation Protection* by Harald H. Rossi (1984) [available also in *Some Issues Important in Developing Basic Radiation Protection Recommendations*, see above]
9	*Truth (and Beauty) in Radiation Measurement* by John H. Harley (1985) [available also in *Radioactive Waste*, see above]
10	*Biological Effects of Non-ionizing Radiations: Cellular Properties and Interactions* by Herman P. Schwan (1987) [available also in *Nonionizing Electromagnetic Radiations and Ultrasound*, see above]
11	*How to be Quantitative about Radiation Risk Estimates* by Seymour Jablon (1988) [available also in *New Dosimetry at Hiroshima and Nagasaki and its Implications for Risk Estimates*, see above]
12	*How Safe is Safe Enough?* by Bo Lindell (1988) [available also in *Radon*, see above]
13	*Radiobiology and Radiation Protection: The Past Century and Prospects for the Future* by Arthur C. Upton (1989) [available also in *Radiation Protection Today*, see above]
14	*Radiation Protection and the Internal Emitter Saga* by J. Newell Stannard (1990) [available also in *Health and Ecological Implications of Radioactively Contaminated Environments*, see above]
15	*When is a Dose Not a Dose?* by Victor P. Bond (1992) [available also in *Genes, Cancer and Radiation Protection*, see above]

16 *Dose and Risk in Diagnostic Radiology: How Big? How Little?* by Edward W. Webster (1992) [available also in *Radiation Protection in Medicine*, see above]

17 *Science, Radiation Protection and the NCRP* by Warren K. Sinclair (1993) [available also in *Radiation Science and Societal Decision Making,* see above]

18 *Mice, Myths and Men* by R.J. Michael Fry (1995)

19 *Certainty and Uncertainty in Radiation Research* by Albrecht M. Kellerer. Health Phys. **69**, 446–453 (1995).

20 *70 Years of Radiation Genetics: Fruit Flies, Mice and Humans* by Seymour Abrahamson. Health Phys. **71**, 624–633 (1996).

21 *Radionuclides in the Body: Meeting the Challenge* by William J. Bair. Health Phys. **73**, 423–432 (1997).

22 *From Chimney Sweeps to Astronauts: Cancer Risks in the Work Place* by Eric J. Hall. Health Phys. **75**, 357–366 (1998).

23 *Back to Background: Natural Radiation and Radioactivity Exposed* by Naomi H. Harley. Health Phys. **79**, 121–128 (2000).

24 *Administered Radioactivity: Unde Venimus Quoque Imus* by S. James Adelstein. Health Phys. **80**, 317–324 (2001).

25 *Assuring the Safety of Medical Diagnostic Ultrasound* by Wesley L. Nyborg. Health Phys. **82**, 578–587 (2002).

26 *Developing Mechanistic Data for Incorporation into Cancer and Genetic Risk Assessments: Old Problems and New Approaches* by R. Julian Preston. Health Phys. **85**, 4–12 (2003).

Symposium Proceedings

No.	Title
1	*The Control of Exposure of the Public to Ionizing Radiation in the Event of Accident or Attack*, Proceedings of a Symposium held April 27-29, 1981 (1982)
2	*Radioactive and Mixed Waste—Risk as a Basis for Waste Classification,* Proceedings of a Symposium held November 9, 1994 (1995)
3	*Acceptability of Risk from Radiation—Application to Human Space Flight,* Proceedings of a Symposium held May 29, 1996 (1997)
4	*21st Century Biodosimetry: Quantifying the Past and Predicting the Future*, Proceedings of a Symposium held February 22, 2001, Radiat. Prot. Dosim. **97**(1), (2001)
5	*National Conference on Dose Reduction in CT, with an Emphasis on Pediatric Patients*, Summary of a Symposium held November 6-7, 2002, Am. J. Roentgenol. **181**(2), 321–339 (2003).

NCRP Statements

No.	Title
1	"Blood Counts, Statement of the National Committee on Radiation Protection," Radiology **63**, 428 (1954)
2	"Statements on Maximum Permissible Dose from Television Receivers and Maximum Permissible Dose to the Skin of the Whole Body," Am. J. Roentgenol., Radium Ther. and Nucl. Med. **84**, 152 (1960) and Radiology **75**, 122 (1960)
3	*X-Ray Protection Standards for Home Television Receivers, Interim Statement of the National Council on Radiation Protection and Measurements* (1968)
4	*Specification of Units of Natural Uranium and Natural Thorium, Statement of the National Council on Radiation Protection and Measurements* (1973)
5	*NCRP Statement on Dose Limit for Neutrons* (1980)
6	*Control of Air Emissions of Radionuclides* (1984)
7	*The Probability That a Particular Malignancy May Have Been Caused by a Specified Irradiation* (1992)
8	*The Application of ALARA for Occupational Exposures* (1999)
9	*Extension of the Skin Dose Limit for Hot Particles to Other External Sources of Skin Irradiation* (2001)

Other Documents

The following documents of the NCRP were published outside of the NCRP report, commentary and statement series:

Somatic Radiation Dose for the General Population, Report of the Ad Hoc Committee of the National Council on Radiation Protection and Measurements, 6 May 1959, Science **131** (3399), February 19, 1960, 482–486

Dose Effect Modifying Factors in Radiation Protection, Report of Subcommittee M-4 (Relative Biological Effectiveness) of the National Council on Radiation Protection and Measurements, Report BNL 50073 (T-471) (1967) Brookhaven National Laboratory (National Technical Information Service, Springfield, Virginia)

Index